MARY QUANT ✿

CLASSIC MAKE-UP & BEAUTY

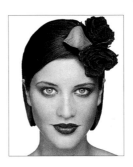

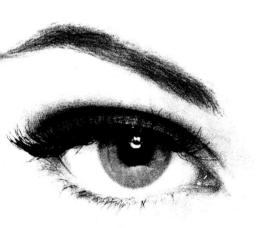
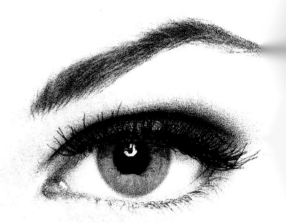
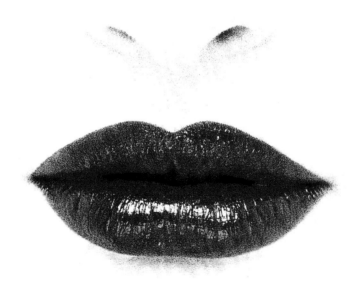

MARY QUANT ❀
CLASSIC MAKE-UP & BEAUTY

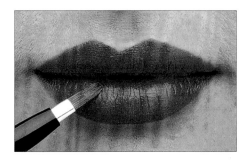

PHOTOGRAPHY
MAUREEN BARRYMORE
DAVE KING

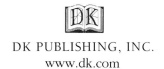

DK PUBLISHING, INC.
www.dk.com

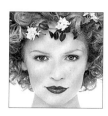

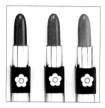

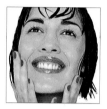

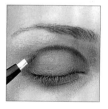

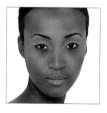

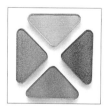

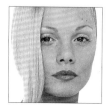

A DK PUBLISHING BOOK
www.dk.com

Project Editor Louise Elliott
Art Editor Helen Diplock
US Editor Laaren Brown
Designer Annette O'Sullivan

Model Photography Direction Michele Walker

Managing Editor Susannah Marriott
Deputy Art Director Carole Ash

Production Manager Maryann Rogers

Additional Photography Steve Gorton

Makeup Artist Cathy Lomax

This book is dedicated to
Juichi Nakayama

First paperback edition, 1998

First American Edition, 1996
13 15 17 19 20 18 16 14 12
Published in the United States by
DK Publishing, Inc.
375 Hudson Street, New York, NY 10014

Quant, Mary.
Ultimate makeup and beauty / Mary Quant.
  p. cm.
Includes index.
ISBN 0-7894-3294-3
1. Beauty, Personal. 2. Cosmetics. 3. Skin-care and hygiene. I. Title.
RA778.Q834 1996   96-2373
646.7'--dc20   CIP

Reproduced by Colourscan, Singapore
Printed and bound in Singapore by Star Standard Industries (Pte.) Ltd.

CONTENTS

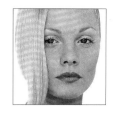

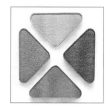
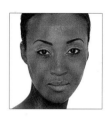
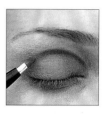
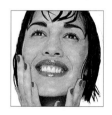
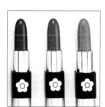
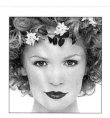

INTRODUCTION

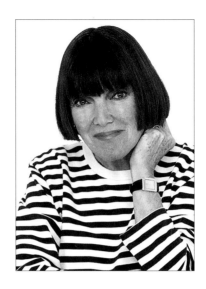

THE POWER OF MAKEUP

Makeup has the power to put you in the mood for whatever lies ahead. It can make you more the person you want to be, and help you feel more at ease or pleased with yourself before launching into the fracas or fun to come. If you are happy with your makeup, you can forget about it and simply get on with life and the pleasure of being you.

I have always been fascinated by the effect of makeup and color on the face. We are often afraid of changing our lipstick or eyeshadow color, but to do so is a way of following fashion as it evolves. I am a believer in experimenting with color: Sometimes a new approach can create the most successful results, and this book will help you to choose and mix color palettes with ease.

DISCOVER THE NEW YOU

Style in makeup is something to explore. Try not to see your makeup as a form of camouflage; instead, use it as a way to bring out the best in your face and even as a way of showing another side of your personality, possibly one you never knew you had. Sometimes glamorous, sometimes pretty, sometimes as natural as can be, the choice is as wide as you want to make it, and a collection of different looks is included here to inspire you.

THE TRICKS OF THE TRADE

Even if you have the best eye for fashion and color and the cleverest ideas for creating stylish new looks, the finished effect is more likely to be brash than beautiful if you do not know how to apply your makeup properly. But if you spend some time in front of the mirror practicing the ground rules and acquiring the tricks of the trade, as revealed in the step-by-step makeup lessons, you will soon be running your liquid eyeliner along in one quick move, sculpting your cheekbones with nothing but a delicate sweep of blusher, outlining your lips to perfection, even applying a pair of false eyelashes with ease.

LAYING THE FOUNDATIONS

To be really successful, makeup must be applied to as clean and healthy a foundation as possible. That is why it is so important to follow a skin-care program and to be aware of the needs of your skin type; both are explained fully in the pages that follow. You should also try to supplement your program as often as you can with a deep-cleansing treatment, such as a soothing face pack. And do not stop at the face – pamper your body, too, with everything from a long, warm bath to a firming massage. Make time every day to spend on yourself so that you look and feel your very best. This book is loaded with ideas to show you how. But remember – rules are made to be broken.

Mary Quant.

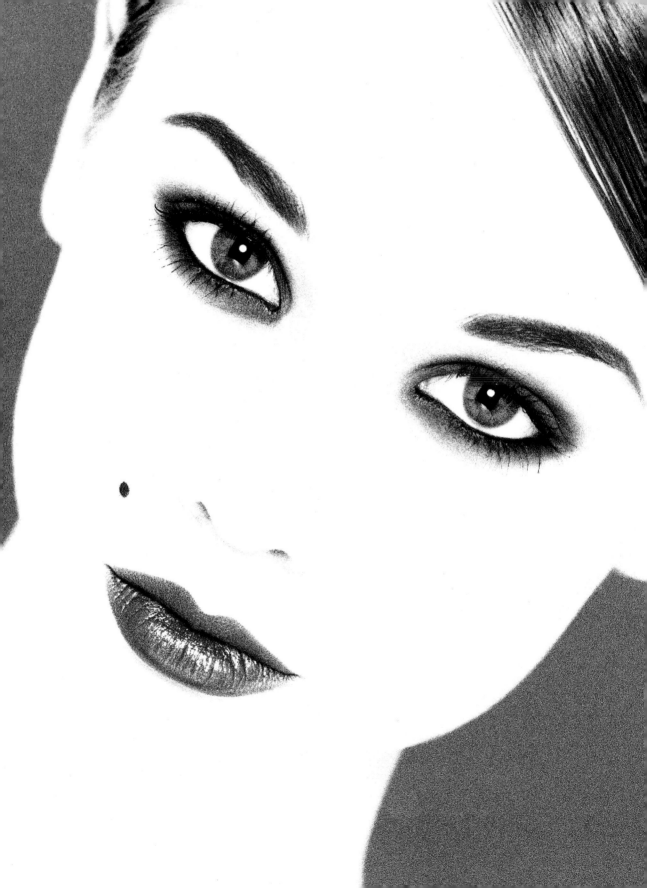

A Gallery of Looks

From dramatic evening glamour to barely-there natural beauty, a wide range of looks can be achieved with clever makeup alone. Here, I have chosen eight different styles to suit every occasion and every mood. And to help you re-create each one, step-by-step instructions explain how to build up to the finished look, while a visual guide reveals all the cosmetics that you will need. Once you feel confident enough, try devising your own looks, drawing on past and present fashions for inspiration.

ICE MAIDEN

The key to this cool, strong daytime look is the clever blending of pearly, pale eyeshadows. White, lilac, pink, and coral work together to create a frosty, shimmering feel that is perfect for brightening bleak winter days. A pearly white eyeshadow is also used to highlight the cheekbones and helps enhance the pale, frosted effect. Lashes and brows are gently outlined in soft brown, while the orange lips and light orange blusher make a dramatic contrast and add a hint of summer to the overall effect.

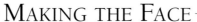

STYLING TIPS

◆ For an extra frosty touch, use a paler foundation than your natural skin tone and add a light dusting of pearly powder to the face, neck, and shoulders.

◆ Do not apply too much eyeshadow all at once: first see how well you can blend the colors together. You can always add more shadow if you want the effect to be stronger.

◆ To complete the shimmering look, choose a nail polish that picks up on one of the eyeshadow colors, such as lilac or pearly pink.

◆ This is a fairly sophisticated look that needs simple but dramatic clothing – anything in silver, black, or midnight blue would increase the impact of the makeup.

MAKING THE FACE

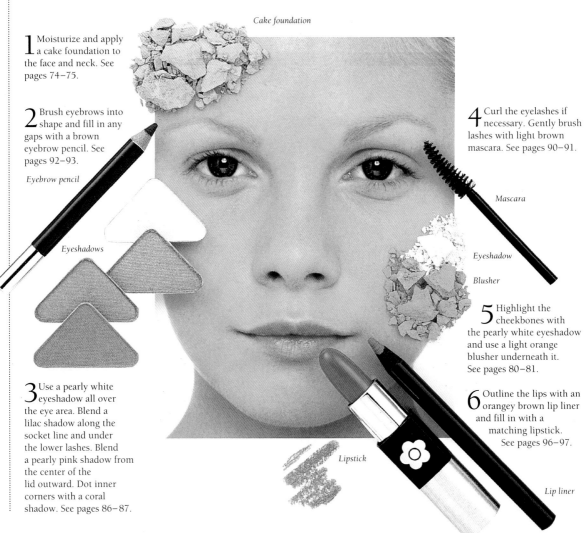

Cake foundation

1 Moisturize and apply a cake foundation to the face and neck. See pages 74–75.

2 Brush eyebrows into shape and fill in any gaps with a brown eyebrow pencil. See pages 92–93.

Eyebrow pencil

Eyeshadows

3 Use a pearly white eyeshadow all over the eye area. Blend a lilac shadow along the socket line and under the lower lashes. Blend a pearly pink shadow from the center of the lid outward. Dot inner corners with a coral shadow. See pages 86–87.

4 Curl the eyelashes if necessary. Gently brush lashes with light brown mascara. See pages 90–91.

Mascara

Eyeshadow

Blusher

5 Highlight the cheekbones with the pearly white eyeshadow and use a light orange blusher underneath it. See pages 80–81.

6 Outline the lips with an orangey brown lip liner and fill in with a matching lipstick. See pages 96–97.

Lipstick

Lip liner

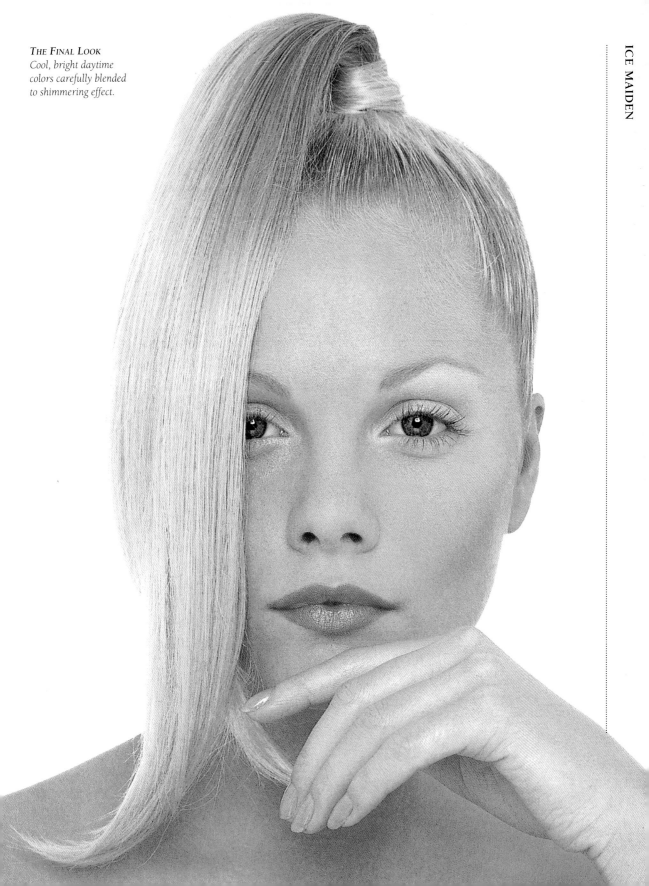

THE FINAL LOOK
Cool, bright daytime colors carefully blended to shimmering effect.

SIXTIES STYLE

Distinctive dark, smoky eyes and pale-colored lips re-create the mood of the 1960s and the stylish mod look for which Mary Quant is so well known. However, this dramatic eye makeup is definitely not for the faint-hearted. Charcoal shadow practically encircles the eyes, while the top and bottom lashes are lined for emphasis and thoroughly coated with black mascara. The smooth-finished base helps accentuate the smoldering eyes, and a light dusting of blusher gives the barest hint of a healthy glow.

STYLING TIPS

◆ For an even more dramatic contrast, choose a paler lip color, such as white.

◆ Use only a very light dusting of blusher – too much and you will look too healthy for the 1960s style.

◆ Dust loose powder underneath eyes to catch color while applying eyeshadow, then brush off afterward.

◆ A sharp Sixties bob is perfect for this look. Alternatively, try backcombing hair into a more unruly beehive style.

◆ For a complete Sixties look, go for clothes that match – a black polo-neck sweater worn with a monochrome pantsuit or miniskirt, for example.

MAKING THE FACE

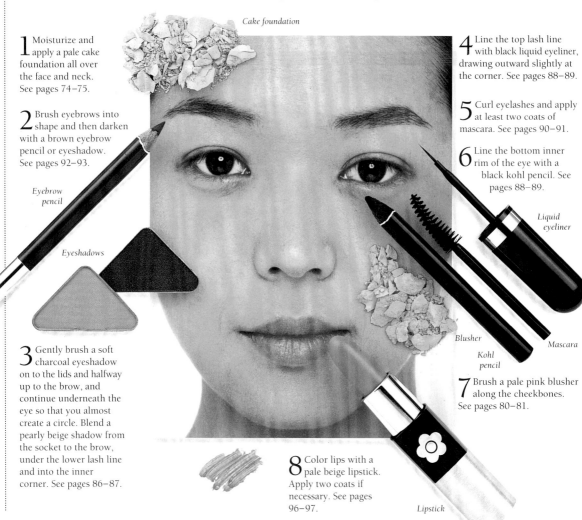

Cake foundation

1 Moisturize and apply a pale cake foundation all over the face and neck. See pages 74–75.

2 Brush eyebrows into shape and then darken with a brown eyebrow pencil or eyeshadow. See pages 92–93.

Eyebrow pencil

Eyeshadows

3 Gently brush a soft charcoal eyeshadow on to the lids and halfway up to the brow, and continue underneath the eye so that you almost create a circle. Blend a pearly beige shadow from the socket to the brow, under the lower lash line and into the inner corner. See pages 86–87.

4 Line the top lash line with black liquid eyeliner, drawing outward slightly at the corner. See pages 88–89.

5 Curl eyelashes and apply at least two coats of mascara. See pages 90–91.

6 Line the bottom inner rim of the eye with a black kohl pencil. See pages 88–89.

Liquid eyeliner

Blusher

Kohl pencil

Mascara

7 Brush a pale pink blusher along the cheekbones. See pages 80–81.

8 Color lips with a pale beige lipstick. Apply two coats if necessary. See pages 96–97.

Lipstick

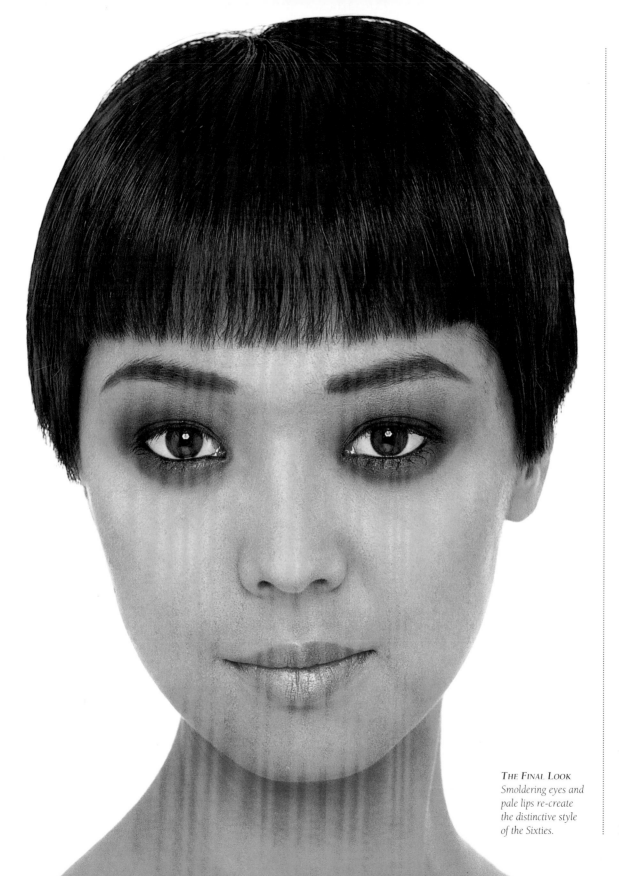

THE FINAL LOOK
*Smoldering eyes and
pale lips re-create
the distinctive style
of the Sixties.*

13

NEARLY NATURAL

The nearly natural or "barely there" look is possibly one of the hardest to achieve. It requires a light, skillful touch and very careful choice of color. The goal is to give the complexion a healthy glow by using foundation and blusher that subtly enhance natural skin tone rather than disguising it, with blusher perfectly blended into the base. Eyelashes have been given only the lightest touch of mascara, and lips the barest brushing of lipstick. Eyeshadow colors follow the rosy pink theme of the blusher.

STYLING TIPS

◆ *Brush eyelashes through carefully with an eyelash comb to make sure that lashes do not clump together.*

◆ *Nails should be squarish in shape and not too long. Coat with a clear or light pinky beige polish.*

◆ *Choose a foundation with a sunscreen or added moisturizer*

for extra healthy effect, or wear a tinted moisturizer on its own.

◆ *Team with clothes made from natural fabrics, such as cotton and linen, to continue the fresh theme.*

◆ *Accentuate the natural look with hair that looks sleek, shiny, and healthy.*

MAKING THE FACE

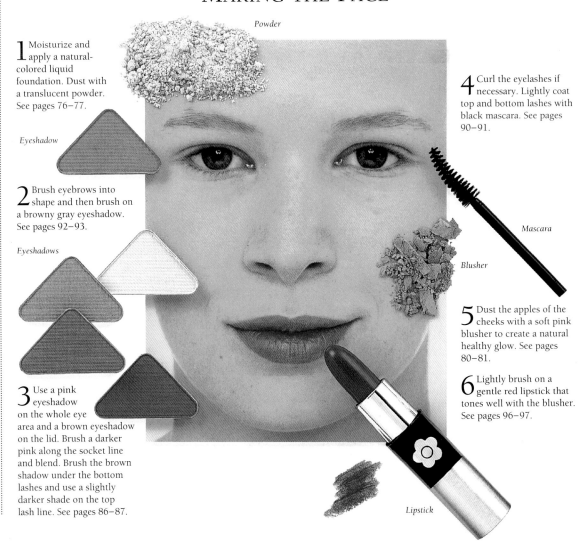

Powder

Eyeshadow

Eyeshadows

Mascara

Blusher

Lipstick

1 Moisturize and apply a natural-colored liquid foundation. Dust with a translucent powder. See pages 76–77.

2 Brush eyebrows into shape and then brush on a browny gray eyeshadow. See pages 92–93.

3 Use a pink eyeshadow on the whole eye area and a brown eyeshadow on the lid. Brush a darker pink along the socket line and blend. Brush the brown shadow under the bottom lashes and use a slightly darker shade on the top lash line. See pages 86–87.

4 Curl the eyelashes if necessary. Lightly coat top and bottom lashes with black mascara. See pages 90–91.

5 Dust the apples of the cheeks with a soft pink blusher to create a natural healthy glow. See pages 80–81.

6 Lightly brush on a gentle red lipstick that tones well with the blusher. See pages 96–97.

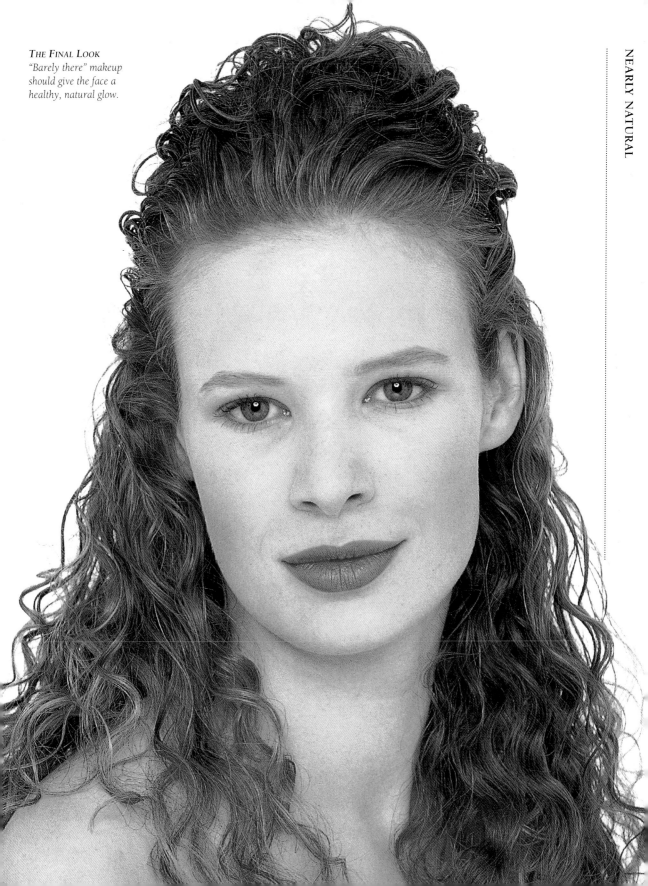

THE FINAL LOOK
*"Barely there" makeup
should give the face a
healthy, natural glow.*

Autumn Glamour

A palette of rich fall colors creates this soft but decidedly glamorous look. Suitable for day and evening, it is based on subtle textures and clever shading, using plenty of dark plums and dusky pinks. Eyes are soft, smudgy, and warm, lips are dark, sensual, and full – perfectly balanced by a warm-toned base and a plum blusher. To complete the effect, choose an accessory that enhances the hair and also blends with and supports the mood of the makeup, such as these dried roses.

STYLING TIPS

◆ Smudge eyeshadows to create a softer, richer look.

◆ Choose an eyebrow pencil that is nearest to your natural shade, and if you are shaping your eyebrows, always pluck from underneath.

◆ Use two coats of mascara to give eyes a darker, more sultry effect.

◆ To enhance the look, choose clothes in the same rich colors – anything in velvet would work especially well.

◆ For extra sparkle, add some shiny accessories such as a diamanté hair clip or necklace.

◆ Avoid severe, tightly drawn hair styles; choose a soft look that gently frames the face.

MAKING THE FACE

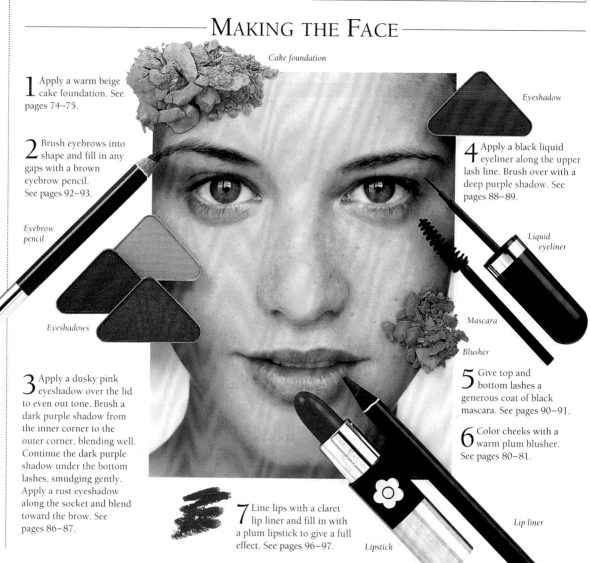

1 Apply a warm beige cake foundation. See pages 74–75.

2 Brush eyebrows into shape and fill in any gaps with a brown eyebrow pencil. See pages 92–93.

3 Apply a dusky pink eyeshadow over the lid to even out tone. Brush a dark purple shadow from the inner corner to the outer corner, blending well. Continue the dark purple shadow under the bottom lashes, smudging gently. Apply a rust eyeshadow along the socket and blend toward the brow. See pages 86–87.

4 Apply a black liquid eyeliner along the upper lash line. Brush over with a deep purple shadow. See pages 88–89.

5 Give top and bottom lashes a generous coat of black mascara. See pages 90–91.

6 Color cheeks with a warm plum blusher. See pages 80–81.

7 Line lips with a claret lip liner and fill in with a plum lipstick to give a full effect. See pages 96–97.

Cake foundation

Eyeshadow

Eyebrow pencil

Eyeshadows

Liquid eyeliner

Mascara

Blusher

Lip liner

Lipstick

THE FINAL LOOK
Very dramatic, this style would be perfect for theater trips or glamorous dinner parties.

PRETTY FACE

Pretty pastel colors are combined for a soft yet striking look that is perfect for midsummer makeup. The really good news about pastels is that they are much easier to apply than the stronger, more definite eyeshadow colors, such as brown or charcoal. Here, the lilacs and blues used around the eyes are beautifully balanced by soft pink lips and a light dusting of pink blusher on the apples of the cheeks. Eyebrows are neatly arched to help open up the eye area and so show off the delicate pastel shades even more.

MAKING THE FACE

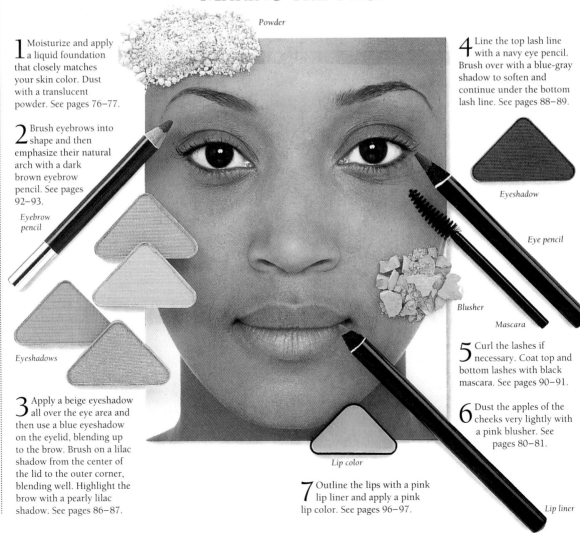

Powder

1 Moisturize and apply a liquid foundation that closely matches your skin color. Dust with a translucent powder. See pages 76–77.

2 Brush eyebrows into shape and then emphasize their natural arch with a dark brown eyebrow pencil. See pages 92–93.

Eyebrow pencil

Eyeshadows

3 Apply a beige eyeshadow all over the eye area and then use a blue eyeshadow on the eyelid, blending up to the brow. Brush on a lilac shadow from the center of the lid to the outer corner, blending well. Highlight the brow with a pearly lilac shadow. See pages 86–87.

4 Line the top lash line with a navy eye pencil. Brush over with a blue-gray shadow to soften and continue under the bottom lash line. See pages 88–89.

Eyeshadow

Eye pencil

Blusher

Mascara

5 Curl the lashes if necessary. Coat top and bottom lashes with black mascara. See pages 90–91.

6 Dust the apples of the cheeks very lightly with a pink blusher. See pages 80–81.

Lip color

7 Outline the lips with a pink lip liner and apply a pink lip color. See pages 96–97.

Lip liner

THE FINAL LOOK
*Pretty pastel colors gently
blended together give a soft
but striking effect.*

FORTIES GLITZ

S trong eyeliner, matte makeup, and rich red lips set a sophisticated and elegant style that draws on the 1940s for inspiration. The shape of the face is given greater definition by highlighting features to create a more sculpted look. Eyebrows are neatly arched to emphasize the sleekness of the eyeliner, and clever use of blusher makes the cheekbones look high and perfectly defined. This look works well for evenings because it gives features greater emphasis and has a dreamy nostalgic feel.

— STYLING TIPS —

◆ *Do not compromise on the strong red lipstick – a lighter color would draw attention away from the mouth and make the eyes look too heavy.*

◆ *Always allow mascara to dry between coats or you will not be able to build up enough color.*

◆ *If you use a concealer, make sure it blends with the base.*

◆ *For extra impact, wear clothes with a 1940s feel, such as an elegant fitted suit, or a classic twin set and A-line skirt or dress. Clip-on earrings or a simple pearl necklace will add to the overall effect.*

◆ *If you do not have wavy hair, try curling it with a curling iron and then brushing through to leave a gentle wave.*

— MAKING THE FACE —

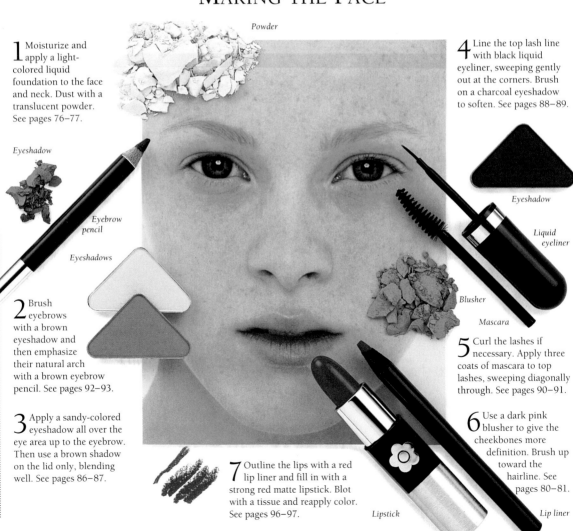

Powder

1 Moisturize and apply a light-colored liquid foundation to the face and neck. Dust with a translucent powder. See pages 76–77.

Eyeshadow

Eyebrow pencil

Eyeshadows

2 Brush eyebrows with a brown eyeshadow and then emphasize their natural arch with a brown eyebrow pencil. See pages 92–93.

3 Apply a sandy-colored eyeshadow all over the eye area up to the eyebrow. Then use a brown shadow on the lid only, blending well. See pages 86–87.

7 Outline the lips with a red lip liner and fill in with a strong red matte lipstick. Blot with a tissue and reapply color. See pages 96–97.

4 Line the top lash line with black liquid eyeliner, sweeping gently out at the corners. Brush on a charcoal eyeshadow to soften. See pages 88–89.

Eyeshadow

Liquid eyeliner

Blusher

Mascara

5 Curl the lashes if necessary. Apply three coats of mascara to top lashes, sweeping diagonally through. See pages 90–91.

6 Use a dark pink blusher to give the cheekbones more definition. Brush up toward the hairline. See pages 80–81.

Lipstick

Lip liner

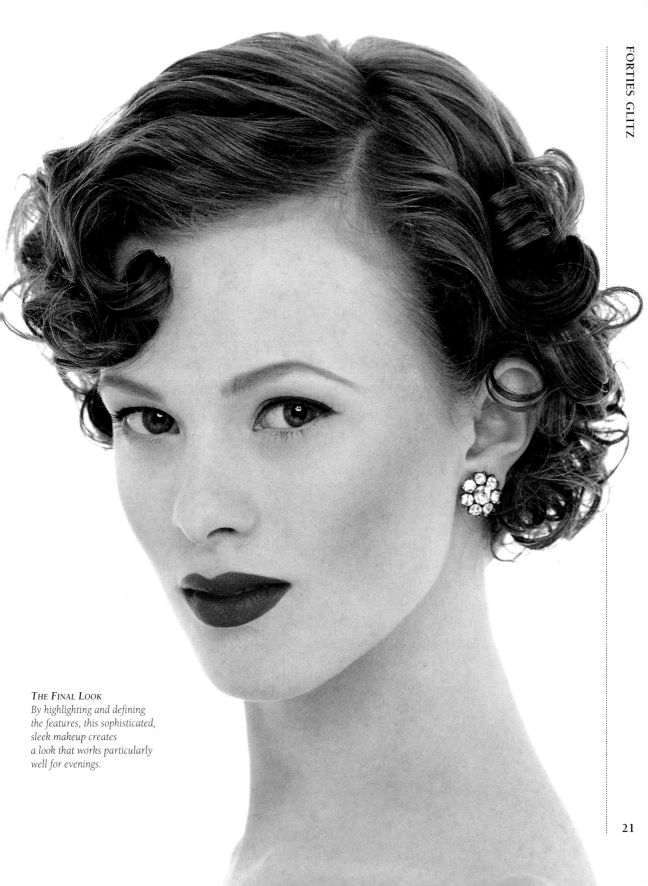

THE FINAL LOOK
By highlighting and defining
the features, this sophisticated,
sleek makeup creates
a look that works particularly
well for evenings.

ACTIVE AQUA

This vibrant, waterproof style is designed for long, hot summer days when you want to spend as much time as possible outdoors and be completely confident that your makeup is not running or smudging. The eye area is brightened and enlarged with a specially formulated eye foundation instead of eyeshadows, and lashes are gently defined with a light coating of waterproof mascara. A hint of cream blusher and strong orange lips add a glamorous touch to an essentially sporty look.

STYLING TIPS

◆ *Before using a waterproof mascara, always check that you have a suitable remover for it.*

◆ *Paint nails in a strong color that either matches or balances the vibrant tone of the lipstick, such as the orange lips and red nails shown here.*

◆ *This is a relaxed daytime effect that suits activewear* rather than anything formal or frilly. Minimize jewelry and accessories; they are not in keeping with this style.

◆ *This type of makeup works well with a sharply cut hair style such as a well-defined boy-cut – avoid anything that might look overstyled. Keep long hair out of the way in a high ponytail.*

MAKING THE FACE

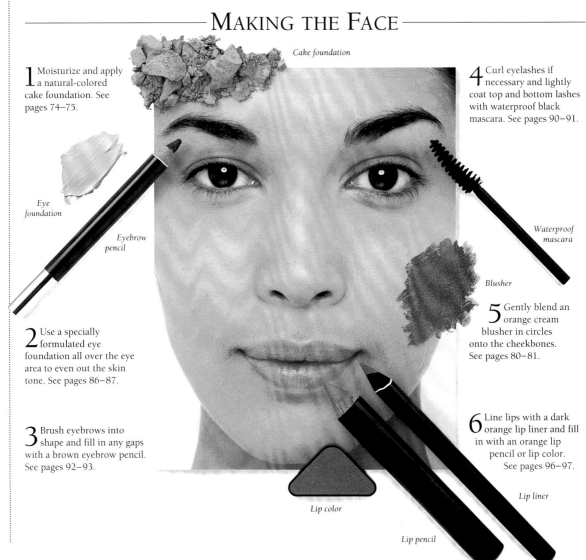

Cake foundation

1 Moisturize and apply a natural-colored cake foundation. See pages 74–75.

Eye foundation

Eyebrow pencil

2 Use a specially formulated eye foundation all over the eye area to even out the skin tone. See pages 86–87.

3 Brush eyebrows into shape and fill in any gaps with a brown eyebrow pencil. See pages 92–93.

4 Curl eyelashes if necessary and lightly coat top and bottom lashes with waterproof black mascara. See pages 90–91.

Waterproof mascara

Blusher

5 Gently blend an orange cream blusher in circles onto the cheekbones. See pages 80–81.

6 Line lips with a dark orange lip liner and fill in with an orange lip pencil or lip color. See pages 96–97.

Lip liner

Lip color

Lip pencil

THE FINAL LOOK
*A strong and sporty
waterproof style to help
you make the most of
hot summer days.*

SPRING BRIDE

A romantic fairy-tale style for those special occasions when you have to look your very best. The secret is a makeup style that is beautiful and bewitching, but never heavy or harsh. Skin looks natural and fresh with just the lightest touch of a pale foundation and a dusting of blusher, while eyes are clear and captivating. The strong mahogany color of the lips strikes an unusual note and introduces a more grown-up edge. Tightly curled locks frame the whole face and help enhance the pre-Raphaelite effect.

STYLING TIPS

◆ Do not be tempted to wear too much mascara; this would make the eyes look too heavy and dark for the fresh, romantic mood.

◆ Try painting nails with green polish to enhance the look of the accessories.

◆ Choosing the right accessories is very important. Keep them as natural and unobtrusive as possible but in keeping with the fairy-tale princess style. Fresh flowers and greenery look great woven into textured hair.

◆ To achieve this hair style, curl hair tightly all over and then brush through, separating curls out slightly. Alternatively, put hair up in a loose bun with gentle tendrils hanging down.

MAKING THE FACE

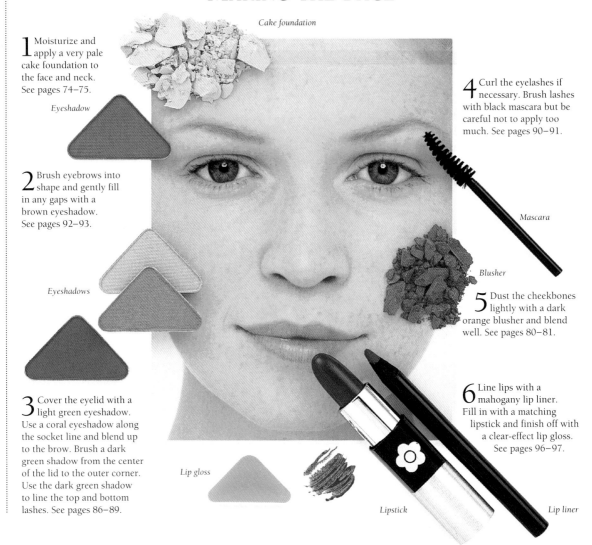

Cake foundation

1 Moisturize and apply a very pale cake foundation to the face and neck. See pages 74–75.

Eyeshadow

2 Brush eyebrows into shape and gently fill in any gaps with a brown eyeshadow. See pages 92–93.

Eyeshadows

3 Cover the eyelid with a light green eyeshadow. Use a coral eyeshadow along the socket line and blend up to the brow. Brush a dark green shadow from the center of the lid to the outer corner. Use the dark green shadow to line the top and bottom lashes. See pages 86–89.

4 Curl the eyelashes if necessary. Brush lashes with black mascara but be careful not to apply too much. See pages 90–91.

Mascara

Blusher

5 Dust the cheekbones lightly with a dark orange blusher and blend well. See pages 80–81.

6 Line lips with a mahogany lip liner. Fill in with a matching lipstick and finish off with a clear-effect lip gloss. See pages 96–97.

Lip gloss

Lipstick

Lip liner

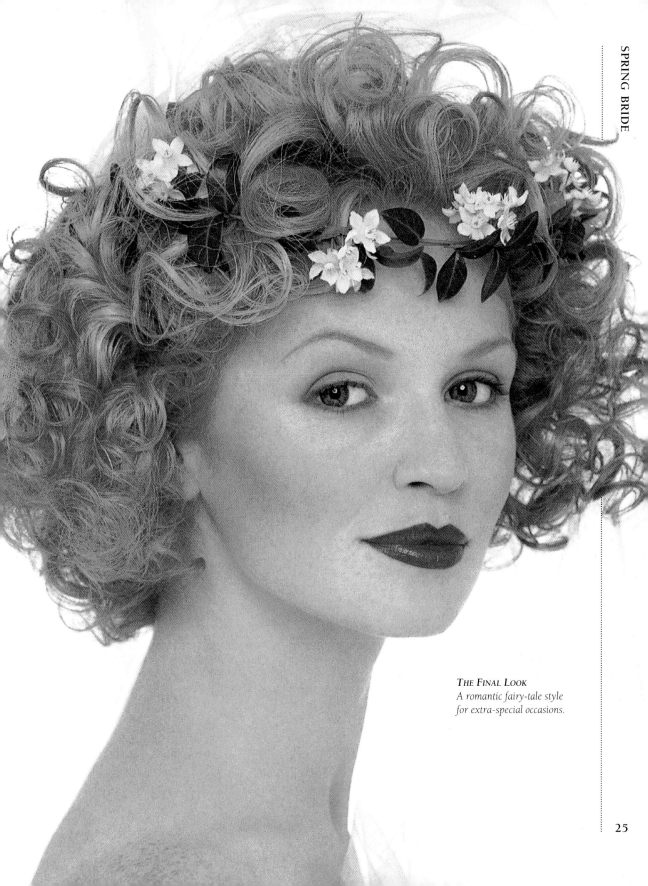

THE FINAL LOOK
*A romantic fairy-tale style
for extra-special occasions.*

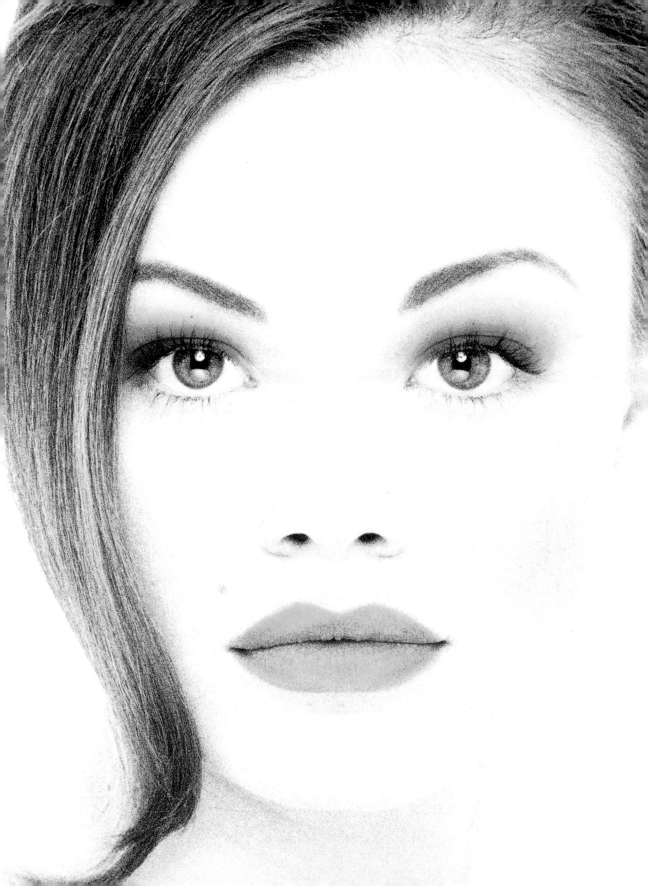

UNDERSTANDING YOUR SKIN

Knowing your real skin type and understanding your true coloring are the first and most important steps you can take toward using cosmetics effectively and making the most of every feature. In this section, easy-to-follow charts, diagrams, and comprehensive color palettes for all types of complexions allow you to find out exactly what makeup will work for you and why. If you get the basics right, you will be well on your way to achieving the very best from your makeup every time.

DISCOVERING YOUR SKIN TYPE

The first, most important step you can take toward caring for your skin properly is to choose the right cleansing products for your particular skin type. The skin on your face is under constant attack from both inside and out, with elements such as the sun and wind causing wrinkles to develop prematurely, and poor diet leading to acne and oiliness. Factors such as stress, pollution, and the changing seasons can also take their toll, making skin look dull, flaky, and lifeless. To combat these enemies, skin needs to be well cared for throughout your life. Moreover, as cleansers, toners, and moisturizers become increasingly sophisticated, it is especially important to use the right one for your skin type. Examine your skin first thing in the morning, then use the chart below to assess which type you are and discover which kinds of products to use and which to avoid.

CHARACTERISTICS OF DIFFERENT SKIN TYPES		CLEANSING
	NORMAL SKIN **Looks:** Clear with an even texture. **Feels:** Soft and smooth. **Problems:** Pimples may occasionally break out, particularly around the chin and nose; dry patches can develop if skin is not cleansed and moisturized.	Use a creamy liquid or cream cleanser, a water-soluble cleanser or gentle facial soap. (See also pages 58–59.)
	DRY SKIN **Looks:** "Thin" or papery with fine pores, and is prone to broken veins on the cheeks. **Feels:** Tight after cleansing, and can react by becoming red and blotchy. **Problems:** Lacks moisture because skin does not produce enough sebum, the skin's lubricating oil. Develops lines more easily than other skin types.	Use a cream cleanser, a very rich liquid cleanser, or a moisturizing, nonperfumed soap, but rinse off thoroughly. (See also pages 58–59.)
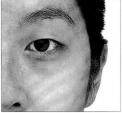	**OILY OR COMBINATION SKIN** **Looks:** Shiny and greasy; combination skin has only patches of oiliness, particularly around the nose, chin, and forehead. **Feels:** Uneven and rough. **Problems:** Prone to pimples, blackheads, and enlarged pores; combination skin may have patches of dryness on the cheeks, as well as acne.	Use a light lotion or a milk cleanser; treat severe skin eruptions with a medicated liquid cleanser. (See also pages 58–59.)
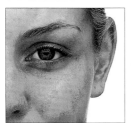	**SENSITIVE SKIN** **Looks:** Clear, but easily becomes red and blotchy. **Feels:** Hot, burning, or stinging when irritated. **Problems:** Reacts when it comes into contact with an allergen or an irritant, either externally or internally; can develop swellings, bumps under the skin, and flakiness.	Use a hypoallergenic cleanser that is free of possible irritants or allergic substances. Avoid using soap, which can strip away the skin's protective layer and so make it more sensitive. (See also pages 58–59.)

THE SKIN'S STRUCTURE

The skin is the body's largest organ and its main function is to provide a protective covering, although it also regulates body temperature and registers touch, pressure, and pain. It is made up of thousands of components, including sweat glands, oil-producing (sebaceous) glands, blood vessels, nerve endings, hair follicles, collagen fibers, fat cells, and sweat pores. The visible skin on the surface of the body is only a small part of this complex organ. Skin has three layers: the epidermis (the top outer layer), the dermis (true skin), and the hypodermis (the bottom layer).

The epidermis is the body's waterproof covering and consists of dead and dying cells that are constantly being replaced by new skin cells formed in the dermis.

The dermis is situated underneath the epidermis and contains most of the skin's living structures, such as blood vessels, nerve endings, and sebaceous and sweat glands. It also includes collagen fibers, which give the skin strength and resilience.

The hypodermis is the deepest layer. It is composed mainly of fat cells, which cushion the blood, lymph, and nervous systems, and help preserve body heat.

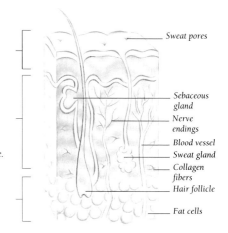

Sweat pores
Sebaceous gland
Nerve endings
Blood vessel
Sweat gland
Collagen fibers
Hair follicle
Fat cells

TONING	MOISTURIZING	TIPS AND CAUTIONS
Use a toner with or without alcohol, rosewater or a still mineral water spray. (See also page 60.)	Use a light cream or lotion, preferably with an added sunscreen. (See also page 61.)	**Tip:** *Normal skin needs just as much attention as dry, oily, or sensitive skin, especially if exposed to extremes of temperature.* **Caution:** *Be careful not to use products that have a tendency to dry out the skin, such as toners with a high alcohol content.*
Use a mild alcohol-free toner, rosewater, or cool water. (See also page 60.)	Use an enriching, protective cream formula, preferably with an added sunscreen. (See also page 61.)	**Tip:** *Pay particular attention to moisturizing, especially the delicate skin around your eyes.* **Caution:** *Check labels to make sure you do not use any products that contain alcohol.*
Use an alcohol-based toner, but avoid those that contain simple alcohols such as ethanol, methanol, and isopropyl – these can be harsh and dry out the skin more. (See also page 60.)	Use a light, non-oily formula, preferably with an added sunscreen; should also be noncomedogenic (it won't block pores). (See also page 61.)	**Tips:** *Moisturize the neck and cheeks thoroughly as these areas can become quite dry; treat pimples with a cleansing stick.* **Cautions:** *Do not be tempted to use harsh cleansers or toners as these will strip away natural oils. Never pick at blackheads or pimples; consult your doctor if acne develops.*
Use a hypoallergenic or alcohol-free toner. (See also page 60.)	Use a hypoallergenic protective cream, preferably with an added sunscreen. (See also page 61.)	**Tip:** *Watch for hypoallergenic cosmetic and sun-care products, too.* **Caution:** *Never use new products without testing them first and waiting 24 hours to see if a reaction develops (see page 59).*

ANALYZING YOUR FACE SHAPE

To use makeup effectively, you need to be aware of the exact shape of your face. Unfortunately, few of us are blessed with the perfect oval and instead fall into the categories of square, heart, round, or long, as well as oblong or triangle, and some of us may be mixtures of these shapes. To analyze your face shape, pull your hair back from your forehead so you can get an overall picture and examine your bone structure carefully in a mirror. Look at your cheekbones, the shape of your jawline and forehead, and the fullness of your cheeks. Pick out your key features and then compare your analysis with the five different face shapes shown here. Once you are aware of the true shape of your face, you can learn how to apply foundation and blusher to create more of an oval outline (see pages 82–83). If you think that your face is a mixture of different shapes, take the key features you can recognize and correct them accordingly (see pages 84–85).

BASIC FACE SHAPES

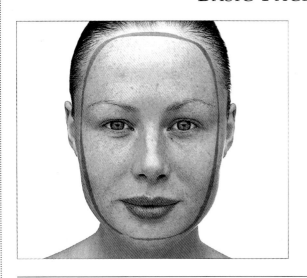

SQUARE

This shape is easily identified by its solid bone structure and square jawline. The forehead is wide and angled, while the cheekbones tend to be flat and unnoticeable. Cheeks often look plump.

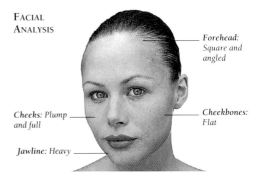

FACIAL
ANALYSIS

*Forehead:
Square and
angled*

*Cheeks: Plump
and full*

*Cheekbones:
Flat*

Jawline: Heavy

HEART

This face is marked by being broad at the top and narrow at the bottom. It can appear long, too, and the chin pointed and prominent. Cheekbones may be high, but often do not show because of the width of the face.

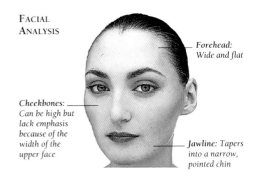

FACIAL
ANALYSIS

*Forehead:
Wide and flat*

*Cheekbones:
Can be high but
lack emphasis
because of the
width of the
upper face*

*Jawline: Tapers
into a narrow,
pointed chin*

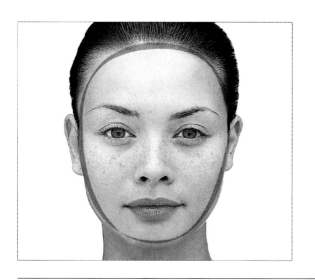

ROUND

Here, the forehead, cheeks, and chin practically form a circle, which can make features look flat and uninteresting. The cheeks are often plump and full, obscuring the cheekbones.

FACIAL ANALYSIS

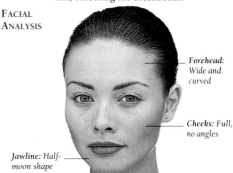

Forehead: Wide and curved

Cheeks: Full, no angles

Jawline: Half-moon shape

LONG

This shape can have either a long forehead or a long chin; features may look drawn and rather raw-boned, creating a tired effect. Cheekbones lack lift because of the length of the face.

FACIAL ANALYSIS

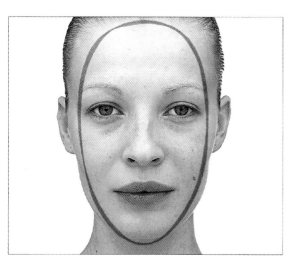

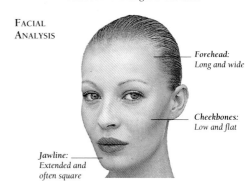

Forehead: Long and wide

Cheekbones: Low and flat

Jawline: Extended and often square

OVAL

The oval face shape has high, sculpted cheekbones with a softly curved jawline that finishes in a delicate chin. The length of the forehead balances the lower part of the face and features look even and neat.

FACIAL ANALYSIS

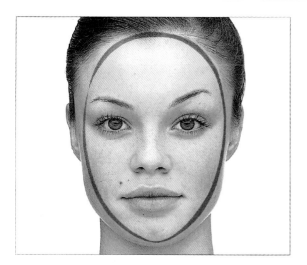

Cheekbones: High and sculpted

Jawline: Gently curved with a delicate, well-defined chin

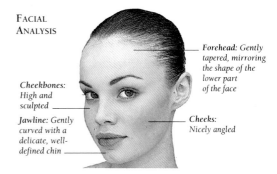

Forehead: Gently tapered, mirroring the shape of the lower part of the face

Cheeks: Nicely angled

31

ANALYZING YOUR COLORING

To ensure foundation looks natural you need to choose a shade that closely resembles your own coloring. Although we all know what color hair we have, we are sometimes surprisingly ignorant about the color of our skin, and choose a foundation just because we like the look of it. Nobody's skin is exactly the same as anyone else's, but we do all fit into distinct groups of color tones: yellow – ivory complexions without much redness; orange – a

mixture of red and yellow; and red – pinkish skin tones without much yellow. Compare your clean skin with the examples shown below to determine which color group you fall into and whether you are pale, medium or dark-toned. Never choose a foundation shade that is outside your own color group, although you can go for a shade lighter or darker depending on the time of year and the effect you want to achieve.

YELLOW TONES

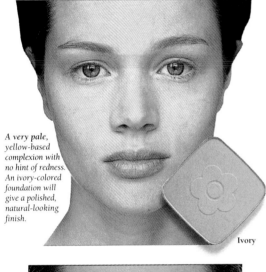

A very pale, yellow-based complexion with no hint of redness. An ivory-colored foundation will give a polished, natural-looking finish.

Ivory

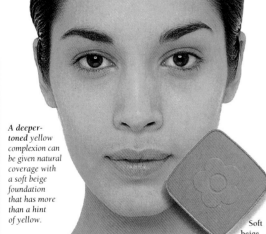

A deeper-toned yellow complexion can be given natural coverage with a soft beige foundation that has more than a hint of yellow.

Soft beige

ORANGE TONES

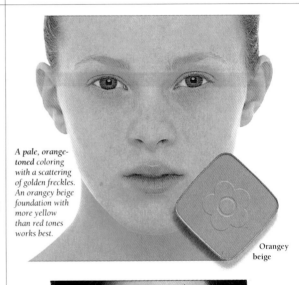

A pale, orange-toned coloring with a scattering of golden freckles. An orangey beige foundation with more yellow than red tones works best.

Orangey beige

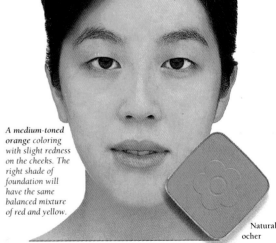

A medium-toned orange coloring with slight redness on the cheeks. The right shade of foundation will have the same balanced mixture of red and yellow.

Natural ocher

32

MATCHING FOUNDATION

When choosing a foundation, always test the color by rubbing a small amount onto a patch of clean skin along your jawline (but not on the wrist, neck, or cheeks as the skin here is a different shade and texture from the rest of your face). Testing foundation along the jawline will also ensure that you do not create a "tidemark" effect between the foundation on your face and the bare skin on your neck. If possible, go out of the store into natural daylight and use a hand mirror to examine the color of the sample foundation; artificial store lighting can alter colors quite dramatically. You should also try to give the foundation time to settle (preferably a few minutes) as some can noticeably change color, particularly on oily skin. The right shade of foundation will "blend" onto your skin, while smoothing out uneven tones and giving you a near-perfect complexion (see pages 74–77). If you want to "lift" your skin tone, wear a foundation that has slightly more pink than your natural shade.

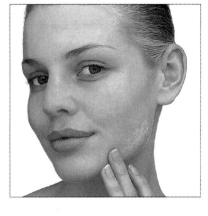

*Test foundation
along the jawline*

ORANGE TONES	RED TONES

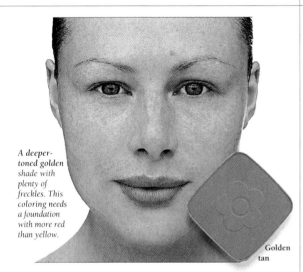

A deeper-toned golden shade with plenty of freckles. This coloring needs a foundation with more red than yellow.

Golden tan

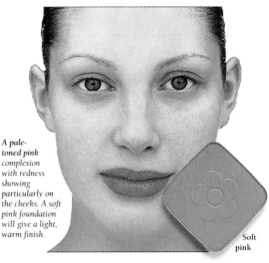

A pale-toned pink complexion with redness showing particularly on the cheeks. A soft pink foundation will give a light, warm finish.

Soft pink

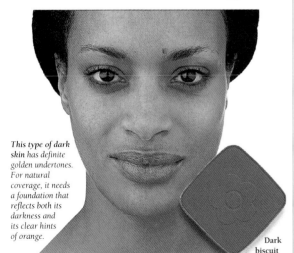

This type of dark skin has definite golden undertones. For natural coverage, it needs a foundation that reflects both its darkness and its clear hints of orange.

Dark biscuit

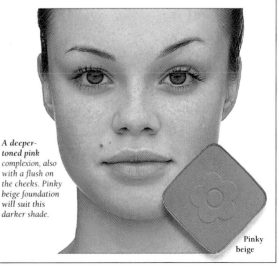

A deeper-toned pink complexion, also with a flush on the cheeks. Pinky beige foundation will suit this darker shade.

Pinky beige

33

CHOOSING COLORS

The crucial point about choosing colors is not to set yourself too many rules – all too often, for example, redheads are told to stick to coppery brown eyeshadows and brown mascara, while those with black skin are usually advised to avoid pinks and blues and to wear nothing but the most muted of lip colors. But this kind of approach to color is limiting; it is only by experimenting with different color palettes – and breaking some of the rules – that you will be able to find the makeup that works best for you and create an exciting range of fresh, new looks (see pages 104–105). The only element for which there is very little room for maneuvering is your foundation, which should always match your natural skin tone as closely as possible (see pages 32–33). To start choosing makeup palettes to suit your natural coloring, take the selections shown here as basic starting points that you can build on and develop according to the different effects you want to achieve.

THE INFLUENCE OF FASHION

Your choice of makeup will also be influenced by the style and color of your clothes. Picking out one bright shade from an item of clothing or jewelry and choosing a highlight eyeshadow to match is an easy way to experiment with more daring colors. Simply dab a little of the color onto the center of the eyelid, smudge, and blend into a neutral-colored base. Because fashion colors are constantly changing, you will need to experiment with new palettes on a regular basis to find the products that work best for you. Styles of makeup change, too. For example, bright lips might be partnered by barely made-up eyes one season, while dark, dramatic eyes and pale, insignificant lips will be the only choice for the next. So to make the most of today's ever-expanding range of makeup colors, you need to keep one eye on what is happening in the fashion world and the other on what suits your natural coloring.

BLACK SKIN

BLACK SKIN

Warm beige, golden brown, burgundy, and terra-cotta are the play-safe choices for black skin. Be more adventurous by creating a contrast with pearly lilacs and bright blues.

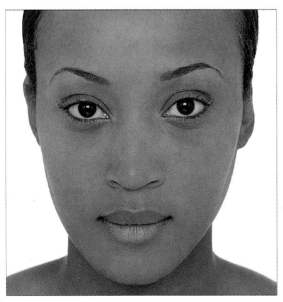

KEY COLORS

BASE

Bronze: *Matches the natural skin tone*

EYESHADOWS

Bright blue and pearly lilac: *For bold, bright impact*

EYELINER

Black eyeliner: *Gives round eyes a sleek look*

MASCARA

Black mascara: *Brings out the beauty of dark eyes*

BLUSHER

Tawny: *A gentle, easy-to-wear color*

Lilac: *Works well with pastel eyeshadows*

Dark red and burgundy: *Deep, warm colors always look good*

LIPS

Mauvey pink: *Looks good with bright or pastel eyeshadows*

Deep burgundy: *Creates a warm, subtle effect*

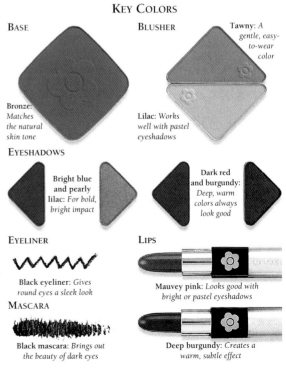

OLIVE SKIN

DARK HAIR/OLIVE SKIN

Complement olive skin and dark brown eyes with warm, deep shades that look strong but natural. Darker mauves, pinks, and blues make an unusual alternative and add extra radiance.

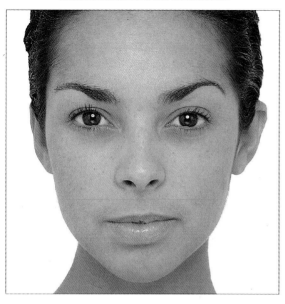

KEY COLORS

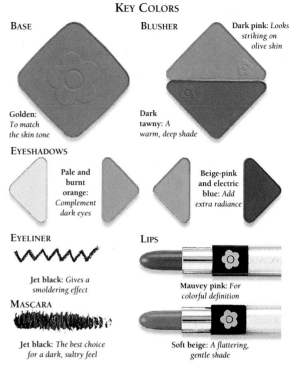

BASE

Golden: *To match the skin tone*

BLUSHER

Dark pink: *Looks striking on olive skin*

Dark tawny: *A warm, deep shade*

EYESHADOWS

Pale and burnt orange: *Complement dark eyes*

Beige-pink and electric blue: *Add extra radiance*

EYELINER

Jet black: *Gives a smoldering effect*

MASCARA

Jet black: *The best choice for a dark, sultry feel*

LIPS

Mauvey pink: *For colorful definition*

Soft beige: *A flattering, gentle shade*

LIGHT BROWN HAIR/OLIVE SKIN

The gold-flecked undertones of light olive coloring are brought to life with warm shades, such as terra-cotta, peach, and soft browns. Pearly lilacs and slate grays are colorful options.

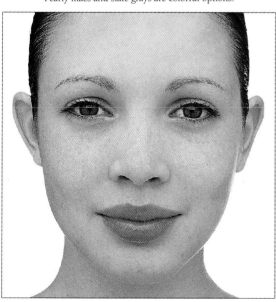

KEY COLORS

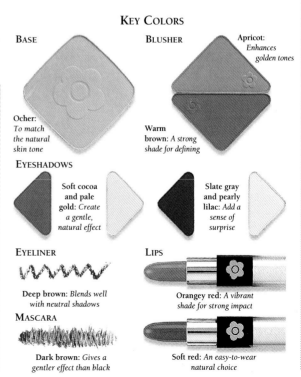

BASE

Ocher: *To match the natural skin tone*

BLUSHER

Apricot: *Enhances golden tones*

Warm brown: *A strong shade for defining*

EYESHADOWS

Soft cocoa and pale gold: *Create a gentle, natural effect*

Slate gray and pearly lilac: *Add a sense of surprise*

EYELINER

Deep brown: *Blends well with neutral shadows*

MASCARA

Dark brown: *Gives a gentler effect than black*

LIPS

Orangey red: *A vibrant shade for strong impact*

Soft red: *An easy-to-wear natural choice*

FAIR SKIN

RED HAIR / PALE SKIN

Pale redheads look good in warm shades that help to enhance their natural creamy tones. But brighter colors can make an exciting contrast, and blue and bronze look good with blue eyes.

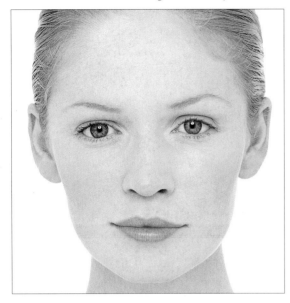

KEY COLORS

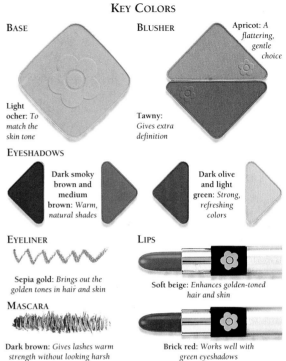

BASE

Light ocher: *To match the skin tone*

BLUSHER

Apricot: *A flattering, gentle choice*

Tawny: *Gives extra definition*

EYESHADOWS

Dark smoky brown and medium brown: *Warm, natural shades*

Dark olive and light green: *Strong, refreshing colors*

EYELINER

Sepia gold: *Brings out the golden tones in hair and skin*

LIPS

Soft beige: *Enhances golden-toned hair and skin*

MASCARA

Dark brown: *Gives lashes warm strength without looking harsh*

Brick red: *Works well with green eyeshadows*

FAIR HAIR / PALE SKIN

Cool-toned makeup, such as a mauvey brown lipstick, is a dramatic option for this coloring, but soft, baby shades work well for a decidedly pretty effect.

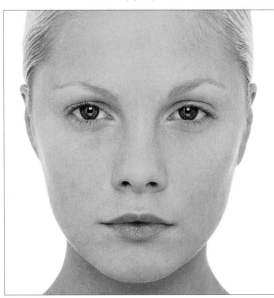

KEY COLORS

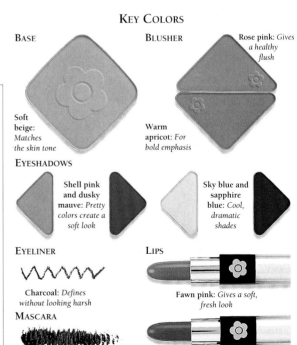

BASE

Soft beige: *Matches the skin tone*

BLUSHER

Rose pink: *Gives a healthy flush*

Warm apricot: *For bold emphasis*

EYESHADOWS

Shell pink and dusky mauve: *Pretty colors create a soft look*

Sky blue and sapphire blue: *Cool, dramatic shades*

EYELINER

Charcoal: *Defines without looking harsh*

LIPS

Fawn pink: *Gives a soft, fresh look*

MASCARA

Black: *Defines and lengthens lashes*

Mauvey brown: *For strong impact*

Asian Skin

BEIGE-TONED ASIAN SKIN

Warm colors, such as apricot and terra-cotta, flatter this kind of coloring. Reflective metallic shades also work well and help lift the face, but they must be perfectly blended. Try to pick up on fashion colors, too.

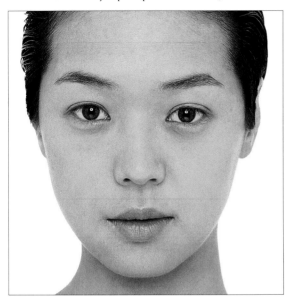

KEY COLORS

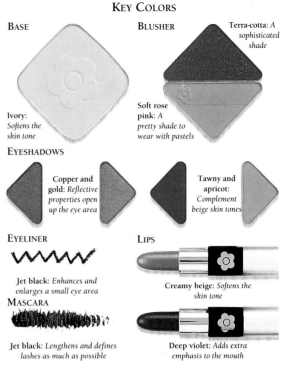

BASE

Ivory: *Softens the skin tone*

EYESHADOWS

Copper and gold: *Reflective properties open up the eye area*

BLUSHER

Terra-cotta: *A sophisticated shade*

Soft rose pink: *A pretty shade to wear with pastels*

Tawny and apricot: *Complement beige skin tones*

EYELINER

Jet black: *Enhances and enlarges a small eye area*

MASCARA

Jet black: *Lengthens and defines lashes as much as possible*

LIPS

Creamy beige: *Softens the skin tone*

Deep violet: *Adds extra emphasis to the mouth*

PALE-TONED ASIAN SKIN

Neutral shades on the eyes and deep color on the lips are the traditional choices for this coloring. Create more modern impact with brighter, vibrant colors, but limit them to the eyes or the mouth.

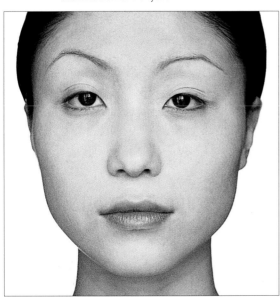

KEY COLORS

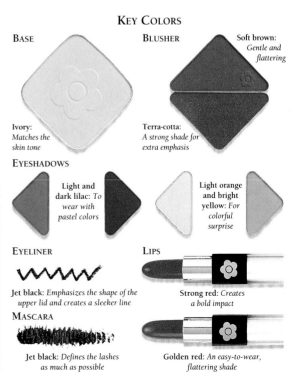

BASE

Ivory: *Matches the skin tone*

EYESHADOWS

Light and dark lilac: *To wear with pastel colors*

BLUSHER

Soft brown: *Gentle and flattering*

Terra-cotta: *A strong shade for extra emphasis*

Light orange and bright yellow: *For colorful surprise*

EYELINER

Jet black: *Emphasizes the shape of the upper lid and creates a sleeker line*

MASCARA

Jet black: *Defines the lashes as much as possible*

LIPS

Strong red: *Creates a bold impact*

Golden red: *An easy-to-wear, flattering shade*

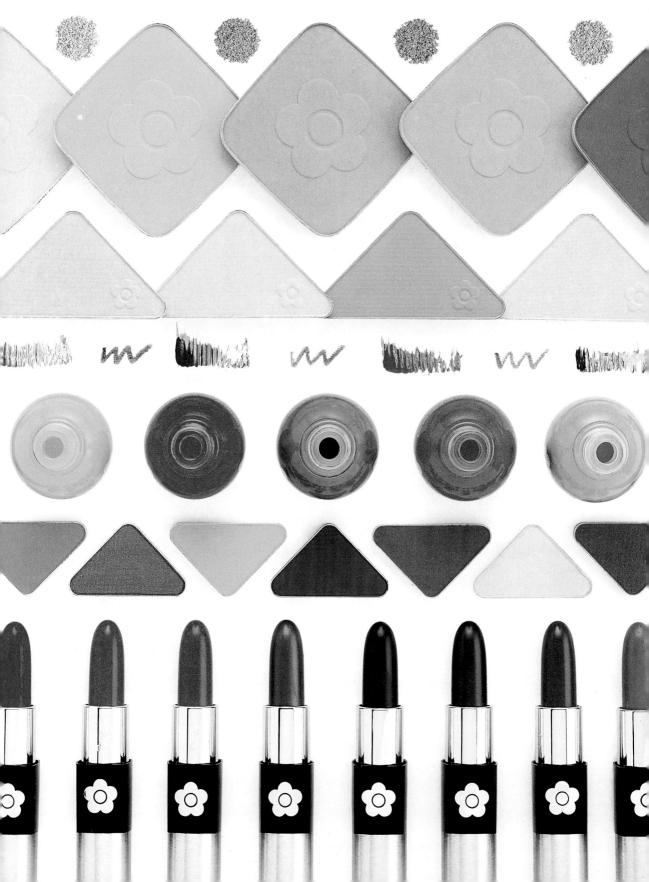

THE MAKEUP
PALETTE

I have always believed that choosing makeup should

be lots of fun, as well as something of an adventure. That

is why I developed a kaleidoscopic range of colors for

eyeshadows, lipsticks, mascaras, nail polishes,

even powders and foundations. To whet your appetite, this

beautifully photographed photo album offers a tantalizing

taste of all the beauty-care products that you can now

choose from, as well as the essential pieces of

equipment that you will need to apply each one properly.

ESSENTIAL EQUIPMENT

You do not need to spend a fortune on your equipment, but having the right tools really does make applying makeup much easier. Using the right sponge will help foundation smooth on more easily and evenly, for example, while having a collection of different-sized brushes will allow you to apply eye and lip colors more easily and blend them where necessary. Store your equipment neatly in a makeup box, or even a tool box, rather than leaving it lying around the bathroom.

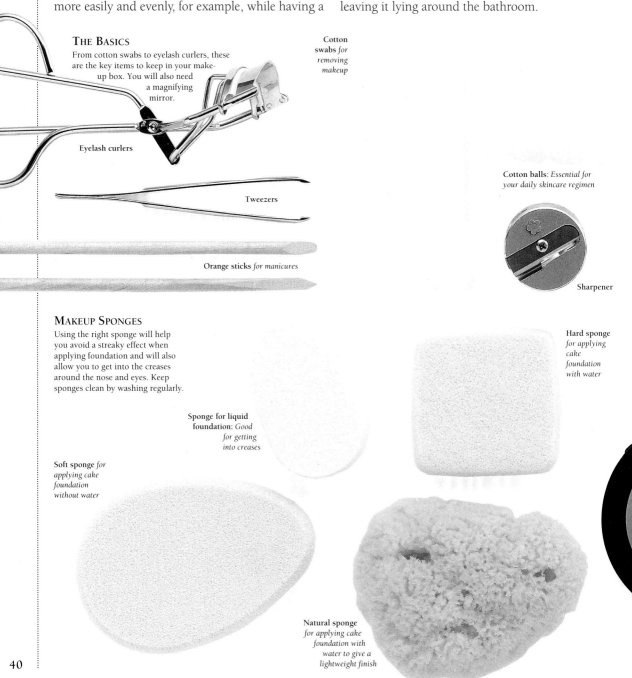

THE BASICS
From cotton swabs to eyelash curlers, these are the key items to keep in your make-up box. You will also need a magnifying mirror.

Cotton swabs *for removing makeup*

Eyelash curlers

Tweezers

Cotton balls: *Essential for your daily skincare regimen*

Orange sticks *for manicures*

Sharpener

MAKEUP SPONGES
Using the right sponge will help you avoid a streaky effect when applying foundation and will also allow you to get into the creases around the nose and eyes. Keep sponges clean by washing regularly.

Sponge for liquid foundation: *Good for getting into creases*

Hard sponge *for applying cake foundation with water*

Soft sponge *for applying cake foundation without water*

Natural sponge *for applying cake foundation with water to give a lightweight finish*

EYESHADOW BRUSHES

A selection of different-sized eyeshadow brushes is essential. Use a large one for applying eyeshadow to the whole eye area and for blending, a medium one for the lids, and a small one for covering the socket line and applying highlighter.

Large eyeshadow brush

Small eyeshadow brush

Soft tip
for blending

Medium eyeshadow brushes

Flexible brush
for eyebrows

BROW BRUSH

This two-in-one tool is ideal for brushing eyebrows into shape and combing out mascara from lashes.

Fine comb
for lashes

Smaller blusher brush *for more controlled blending*

LASH SEPARATOR

Used after mascara has been applied and allowed to dry, this brush separates lashes and prevents clogging.

Spiral nylon wand
to reduce clogging

Large blusher brush

BLUSHER BRUSHES

Use a soft, wide brush to prevent harsh lines and make blending easy, a smaller brush for more controlled blending.

LIP BRUSH

A firm-tipped lip brush gives you greater control over applying color than a conventional lipstick and also allows you to build up a deeper shade.

Lip brush

Powder compact

Powder brush

Powder puff

POWDER APPLICATORS

A soft puff is the perfect way to apply loose face powder. Brush off the excess with a large dome-shaped brush.

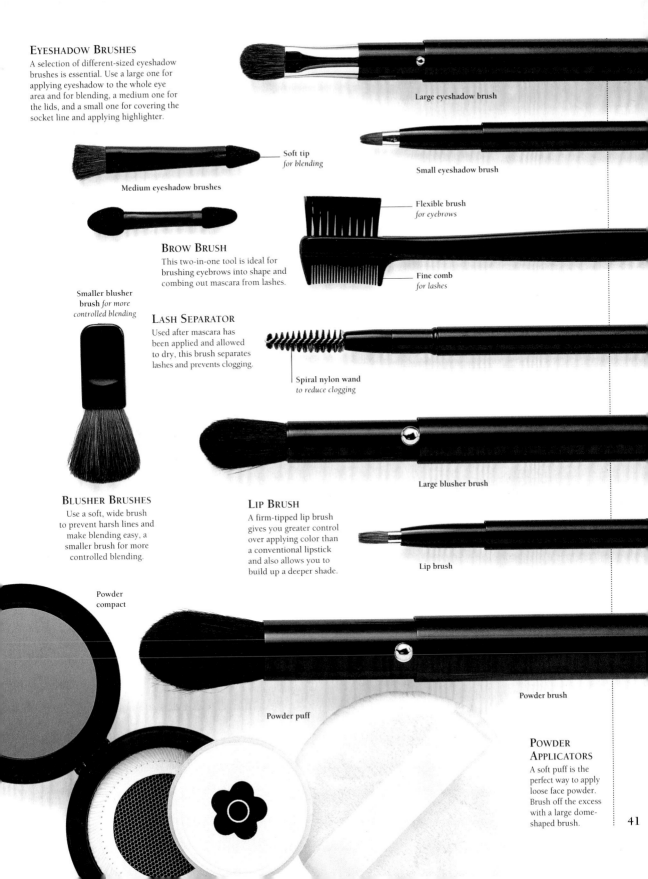

FOUNDATIONS

A foundation should make your skin look as smooth and clear as possible, while also helping to even out the tone. It will then provide the perfect base for the rest of your makeup. Foundations come in a wide variety of colors and types, and it is very important to choose the right one for your coloring (see pages 32–33) and for the effect you want to achieve. For example, in summer you may want the lightest of coverings, while in winter you may prefer heavier protection.

COLOR CORRECTORS

Applied before foundation, color correctors even out specific skin-tone problems. Blue will make a reddish complexion look brighter and whiter; white brightens dull skin and helps cover dark under-eye circles; green will cool down redness; and purple will correct yellowish dullness and add a healthy glow.

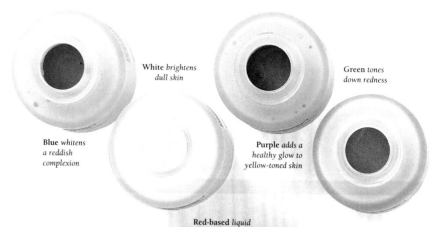

White *brightens dull skin*

Green *tones down redness*

Blue *whitens a reddish complexion*

Purple *adds a healthy glow to yellow-toned skin*

LIQUID FOUNDATIONS

These are usually water-based and can be spread onto the skin easily using a sponge to give lightweight coverage. Always make sure you choose the right one for your skin type – "oil-free" is good for oily skins, while "moisturizing" is better for drier and normal skins. Look for products that also provide protection against the sun's UV rays.

Red-based *liquid foundations suit pink-beige skin tones without much yellow*

Yellow-based *liquid foundations suit ivory-beige skin tones without much red*

Orange-based *liquid foundations suit skin tones with a balanced mixture of red and yellow*

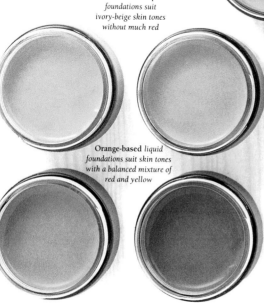

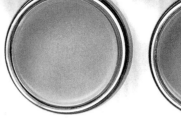

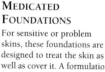

MEDICATED FOUNDATIONS

For sensitive or problem skins, these foundations are designed to treat the skin as well as cover it. A formulation for dry skin, for example, will contain moisturizing agents, while one for very oily skin will include strong oil-controlling ingredients.

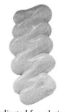

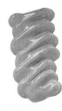

Medicated foundation *for dry skin*

Medicated foundation *for oily skin*

CAKE FOUNDATIONS

Pressed blocks of color, cake foundations generally have a powder element to help control shine. Cake foundations can be applied with either a damp or dry sponge – check the instructions. This type of foundation is good for all skin types and quick to apply. Look for products that help moisturize and protect the skin as well.

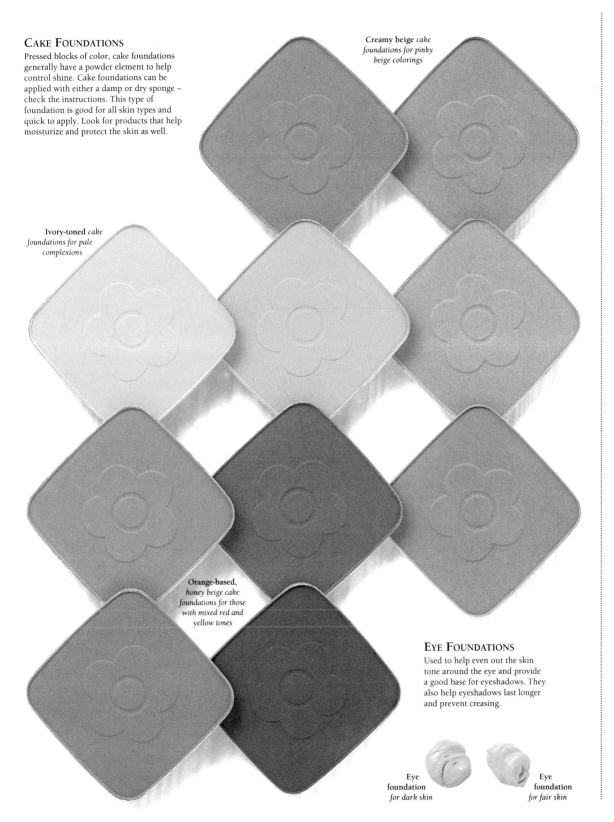

Creamy beige *cake foundations for pinky beige colorings*

Ivory-toned *cake foundations for pale complexions*

Orange-based, *honey beige cake foundations for those with mixed red and yellow tones*

EYE FOUNDATIONS

Used to help even out the skin tone around the eye and provide a good base for eyeshadows. They also help eyeshadows last longer and prevent creasing.

Eye foundation *for dark skin*

Eye foundation *for fair skin*

FACE POWDERS

Powder will add the finishing touch to your foundation and help maintain a fresh, smooth look throughout the day. You can also use powder just on its own for a very natural effect. But whether you are using a loose powder or a pressed powder, never put too much on, and be particularly careful around the eyes, where powder can easily settle into fine lines and so accentuate them. For extra protection, choose a powder that has an added sunscreen or moisturizer.

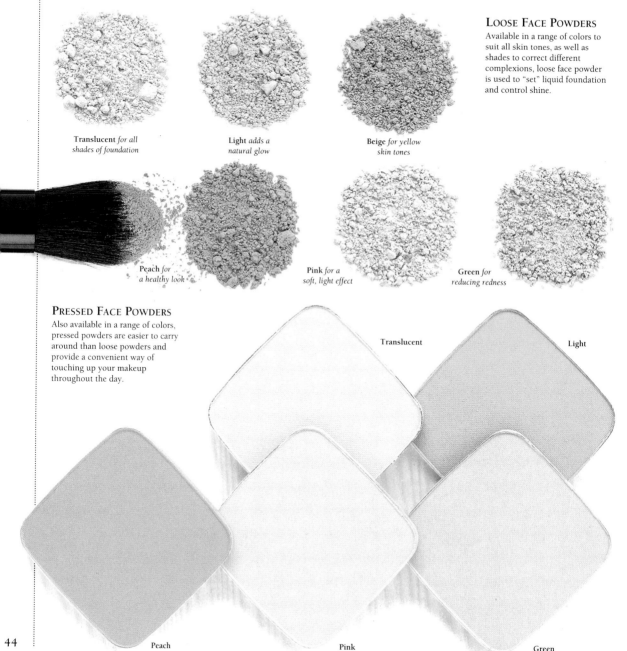

LOOSE FACE POWDERS
Available in a range of colors to suit all skin tones, as well as shades to correct different complexions, loose face powder is used to "set" liquid foundation and control shine.

Translucent *for all shades of foundation*

Light *adds a natural glow*

Beige *for yellow skin tones*

Peach *for a healthy look*

Pink *for a soft, light effect*

Green *for reducing redness*

PRESSED FACE POWDERS
Also available in a range of colors, pressed powders are easier to carry around than loose powders and provide a convenient way of touching up your makeup throughout the day.

Translucent

Light

Peach

Pink

Green

BLUSHERS

Once you know how to apply blusher properly to highlight and define your cheekbones (see Applying Blusher on pages 80–81), it will become an invaluable part of your makeup. Today's blushers contain ultra-fine powder particles to give the skin a natural finish and to prevent harsh lines. Powder blusher is the most popular form as it is the easiest to blend; apply it after foundation but before face powder. Be sure your blusher and lipstick are similar in tone.

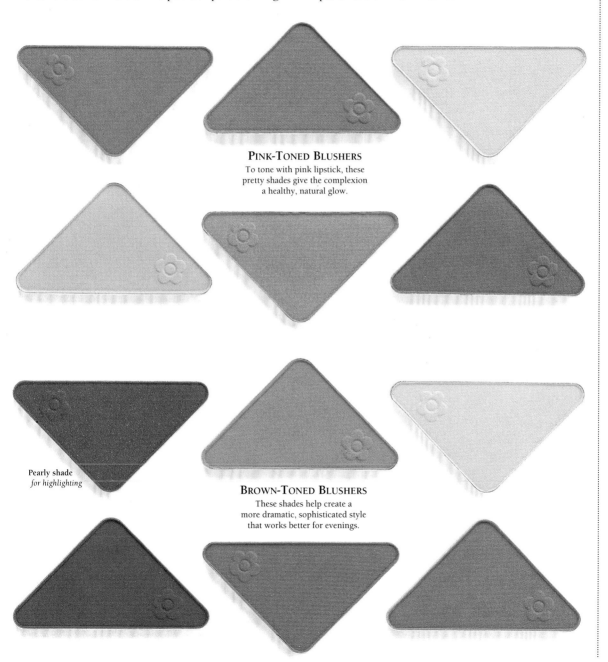

PINK-TONED BLUSHERS
To tone with pink lipstick, these pretty shades give the complexion a healthy, natural glow.

Pearly shade
for highlighting

BROWN-TONED BLUSHERS
These shades help create a more dramatic, sophisticated style that works better for evenings.

EYESHADOWS

Eyeshadows are available in a kaleidoscopic range of colors. However, it is very easy to get stuck in a rut believing that because you have blue eyes you should only use blue eyeshadows. There are no hard and fast rules about which colors should be used with eyes of different colors: try experimenting with new colors, but always use shadows that are within the same color group and complement one another. This will also help you blend and soften the colors easily.

PEARLY SHADES

These are used for highlighting the brow bone to open up the eye area or for creating a shimmering, frosted effect (see the Ice Maiden look on pages 10–11). If your eyelids are particularly crêpey, avoid shadows that are too pearly; they will easily become very creased.

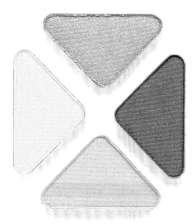

Pearly greens: *Great to wear with taupe, aqua, pale blue, green or white*

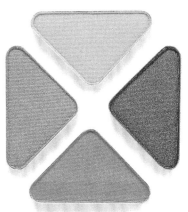

Yellows and oranges *with a pearly finish: Team with citrus colors*

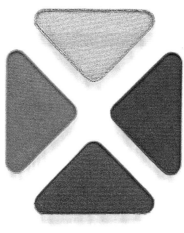

Pearly pinks, reds and violets: *Use to accentuate pale pink clothes, or to lift black and white T-shirts*

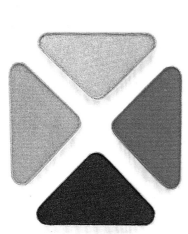

Blues *with a pearly finish: A good choice for jeans, soft blue or black outfits*

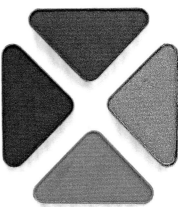

Pearly browns and golds: *Combine with purple or lilac tops to enhance their effect*

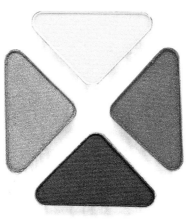

MATTE SHADES

Give a smooth, flat effect. Darker shades help "retreat" eyes, and lighter ones "advance" them. Try blending a dab of pearly eyeshadow on top of a matte shade as a way of experimenting with more adventurous colors (see page 34).

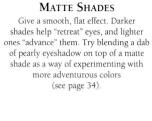

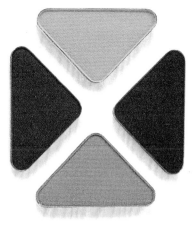

Matte greens: *Cool, sophisticated shades that look wonderful worn with black or white*

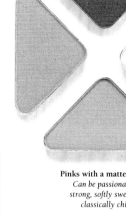

Matte oranges and yellows: *Hot, bright shades work well with vibrant fashion colors*

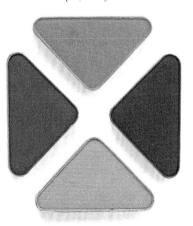

Pinks with a matte finish: *Can be passionately strong, softly sweet or classically chic*

Matte blues and violets: *Lighter shades are pretty and gentle; darker ones deep and moody*

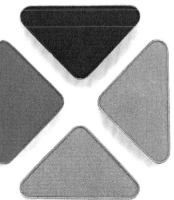
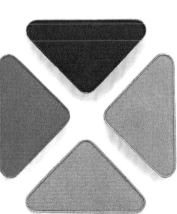

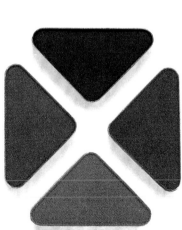

Matte browns: *Soft, neutral colors are ideal for creating sculpted, wide-eyed looks*

Eyeliner & Mascara

Like eyeshadows, eyeliner and mascara help define and enhance your eyes. Eyeliner accentuates the shape of your eyes, while mascara strengthens and darkens the lashes for greater emphasis. They should be the same color, or just a shade lighter or darker, and should mirror each other in shape. For example, eyeliner that sweeps out at the corners looks best when mascara is swept diagonally through the lashes – see the Forties Glitz look on pages 20–21.

EYE PENCILS

These are used to define the top and bottom lash lines, and some can be used inside the bottom inner rim of the eye, too. When using on the top lash line, soften with an eyeshadow.

LIQUID EYELINER

Normally only used along the top lash line, this creates a more intense color than other types of eyeliner. However, it is also more difficult to apply and requires a steady hand.

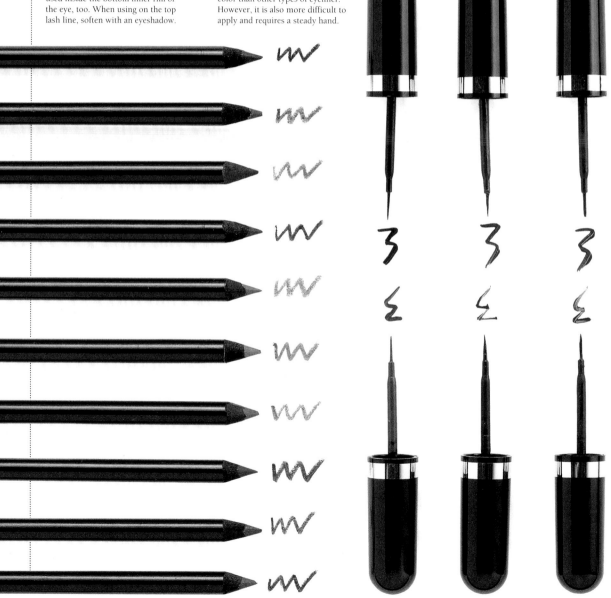

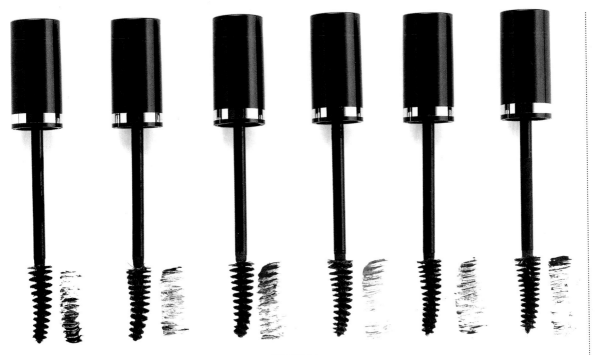

MASCARA

A mascara should thicken and lengthen the lashes without causing them to clump together. Waterproof mascaras are more long lasting but can take longer to remove. Black and brown are the traditional favorites, while more colorful shades can create a bright, dramatic effect.

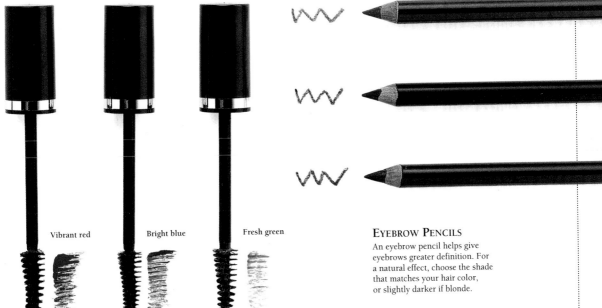

Vibrant red   Bright blue   Fresh green

EYEBROW PENCILS

An eyebrow pencil helps give eyebrows greater definition. For a natural effect, choose the shade that matches your hair color, or slightly darker if blonde.

49

LIP COLORS

Strong reds for sophisticated glamour, barely-there pinks and beiges for natural beauty, or vibrant oranges for sporty style. The color of your lips can change your appearance immediately. Try not to restrict yourself to wearing just one color all the time. Instead, have several choices to suit the effect you want to achieve and for different-colored clothes. Look for lipsticks and lip colors that moisturize and protect your lips, too, and always make sure that they go with your blusher.

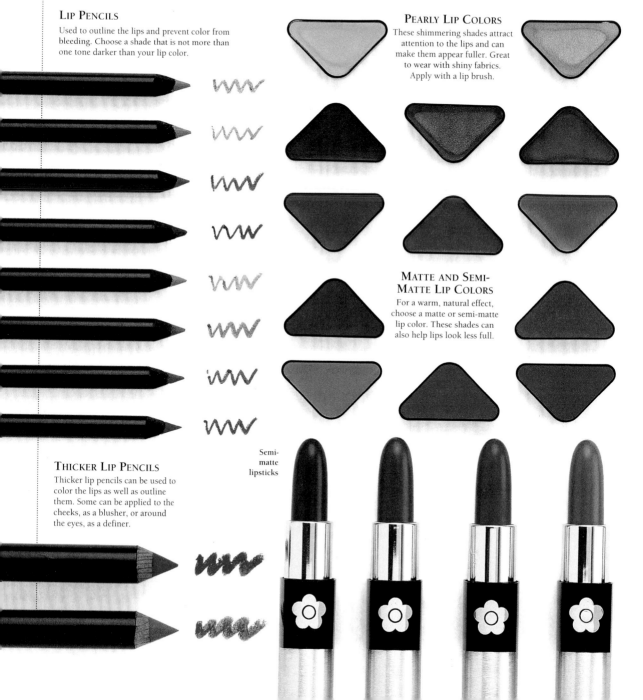

LIP PENCILS
Used to outline the lips and prevent color from bleeding. Choose a shade that is not more than one tone darker than your lip color.

PEARLY LIP COLORS
These shimmering shades attract attention to the lips and can make them appear fuller. Great to wear with shiny fabrics. Apply with a lip brush.

MATTE AND SEMI-MATTE LIP COLORS
For a warm, natural effect, choose a matte or semi-matte lip color. These shades can also help lips look less full.

THICKER LIP PENCILS
Thicker lip pencils can be used to color the lips as well as outline them. Some can be applied to the cheeks, as a blusher, or around the eyes, as a definer.

Semi-matte lipsticks

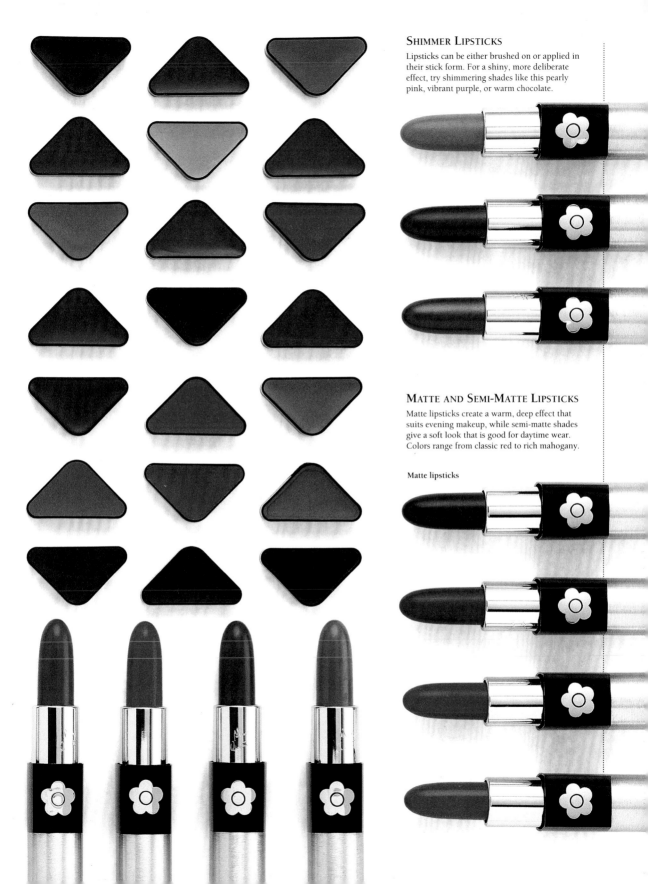

SHIMMER LIPSTICKS

Lipsticks can be either brushed on or applied in their stick form. For a shiny, more deliberate effect, try shimmering shades like this pearly pink, vibrant purple, or warm chocolate.

MATTE AND SEMI-MATTE LIPSTICKS

Matte lipsticks create a warm, deep effect that suits evening makeup, while semi-matte shades give a soft look that is good for daytime wear. Colors range from classic red to rich mahogany.

Matte lipsticks

NAIL POLISHES

Polished nails make the perfect addition to well-cared-for hands, and these days there is a color to suit every mood and every occasion (see Effects for Nails on pages 102–103). Increase the impact of your polish by choosing a color that matches or complements the rest of your makeup, or matches your clothes. Toenails, too, can look fabulous painted with a bright, dramatic color, and not only in summertime. Always remove polish on both hands and feet as soon as it begins to chip.

THE BASICS

For nail polish that lasts well, use a base coat before applying color and finish off with a top coat. Always take off old polish with an acetone-free remover, which will not strip vital oils from your nails.

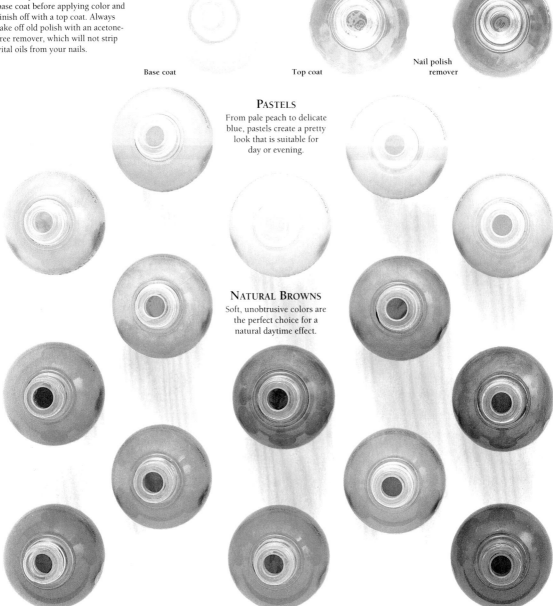

Base coat

Top coat

Nail polish remover

PASTELS

From pale peach to delicate blue, pastels create a pretty look that is suitable for day or evening.

NATURAL BROWNS

Soft, unobtrusive colors are the perfect choice for a natural daytime effect.

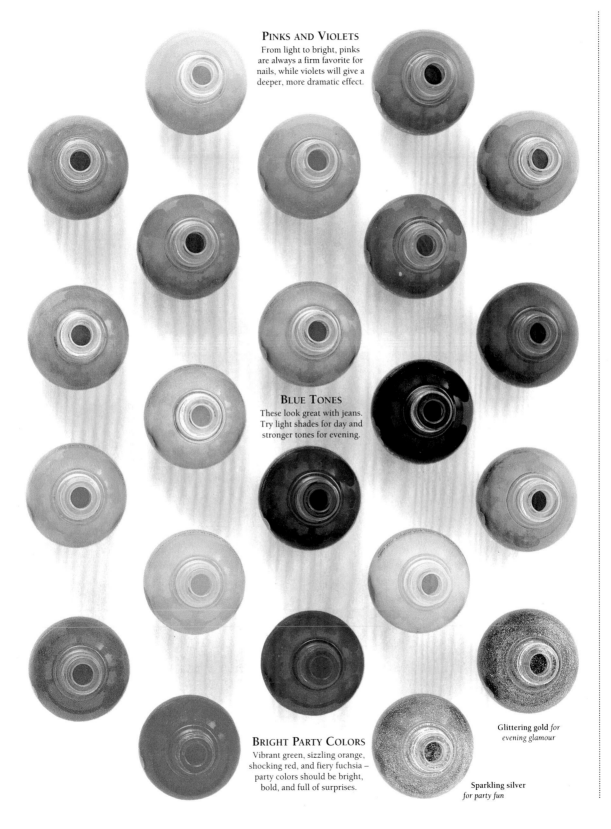

PINKS AND VIOLETS

From light to bright, pinks are always a firm favorite for nails, while violets will give a deeper, more dramatic effect.

BLUE TONES

These look great with jeans. Try light shades for day and stronger tones for evening.

BRIGHT PARTY COLORS

Vibrant green, sizzling orange, shocking red, and fiery fuchsia – party colors should be bright, bold, and full of surprises.

Glittering gold *for evening glamour*

Sparkling silver *for party fun*

SKIN & BODY PREPARATIONS

Young skin is naturally firm, plump, and resilient, but to keep it that way you need to begin a good skin-care regimen as early as possible. Used regularly as a three-step program, cleansers, toners, and moisturizers work together to keep the skin smooth and clear. Really clean skin provides a much better base for makeup, too. The skin on your body also needs frequent attention, and there are now body shampoos, gels, lotions, and scrubs to help you pamper yourself on a daily basis.

CLEANSERS

Cleansers should remove deep-down dirt and makeup without disturbing the skin's balance or stripping away natural oils. Your choice of cleanser will be determined by your skin type (see pages 28–29).

A gentle cleanser *for sensitive and normal skin that cleanses and conditions simultaneously*

A clay-based cleanser *for oily and combination skin that deep-cleanses pores and softens dead skin cells*

An invigorating face scrub *that sloughs off dead cells to leave skin fresh and clean*

TONERS

A toner helps remove any residual traces of cleanser, which could cause irritation, and also helps to make the skin more receptive to moisturizer. After being toned, the skin should feel firm and refreshed but never dry and taut. Look for alcohol-free toners with soothing ingredients, and always use the right toner for your skin type.

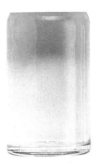

A gentle astringent toner *suits oily to normal skin types*

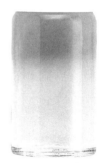

A mild herbal toner *suits normal and combination skin types*

A fragrance-free, alcohol-free toner *suits those with sensitive or dry skin*

MOISTURIZERS

A moisturizer's most basic job is to preserve fluid in the skin's upper layers so that it looks fresh and well hydrated. Whether moisturizers can delay the onset of wrinkles is the subject of debate, but they do help skin to look good. Use a light moisturizer during the day (which will not disturb your makeup) and a richer cream at night when skin can absorb most moisture. If your skin feels dry, treat it to an even richer hydrating cream.

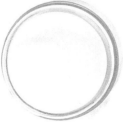

A light gel moisturizer *is good for daytime use and suits all skin types*

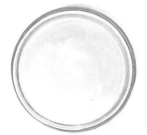

A rich nourishing cream *that will not block the pores is best applied at night*

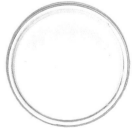

A specially formulated moisturizer *to treat sensitive or dull-looking skin*

BODY CLEANSERS

A warm bath is one of the best places to relax and pamper yourself. Purify the skin with a body shampoo or body scrub, or soak up the soothing properties of a bath oil.

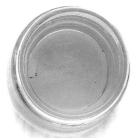

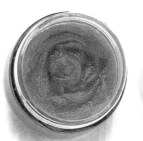

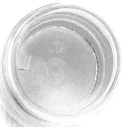

A deep-cleansing body shampoo *that can be easily massaged into the skin*

An extra-fine grained body scrub *to help brush off dead skin cells*

A relaxing bath oil *that leaves skin feeling soft and supple*

BATH CRYSTALS

Make a warm bath even more soothing by adding some fragrant bath crystals with natural ingredients such as sea-water minerals and seaweed extracts.

Rose bath crystals *are gentle and relaxing*

Sea bath crystals *feel fresh and bracing*

Mint bath crystals *are soft and soothing*

BODY MOISTURIZERS

After bathing or showering, massage a non-oily moisturizer all over your body and follow, if desired, with a refreshing lotion, but always use a specially formulated cream to keep hands soft and supple. To combat cellulite, try a special treatment oil or body balm with natural plant extracts.

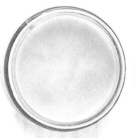

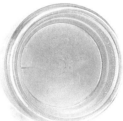

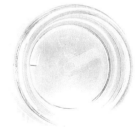

A lightweight, all-over moisturizer *will leave skin smooth and supple*

A refreshing body lotion *to help firm and tone*

A penetrating body balm *to help combat cellulite*

SPECIAL TREATMENTS

In the summer, you may want more protection than an ordinary sun cream can give. A waterproof face block will provide complete protection against the sun's harmful ultraviolet rays, and can also be used as a moisturizing makeup base. As a special addition to your normal cleansing, toning, and moisturizing program, try a deep-cleansing clay face pack to remove deep-down dirt and a hot, firming massage gel to reduce puffiness and bring a healthy glow.

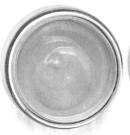

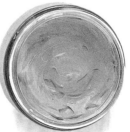

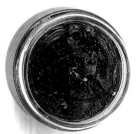

A waterproof sunblock *protects against the sun's harmful ultraviolet rays*

A gentle clay face pack *to help remove deep-down dirt and pollutants*

A heat-promoting gel *that can be massaged into the face and body to reduce puffiness*

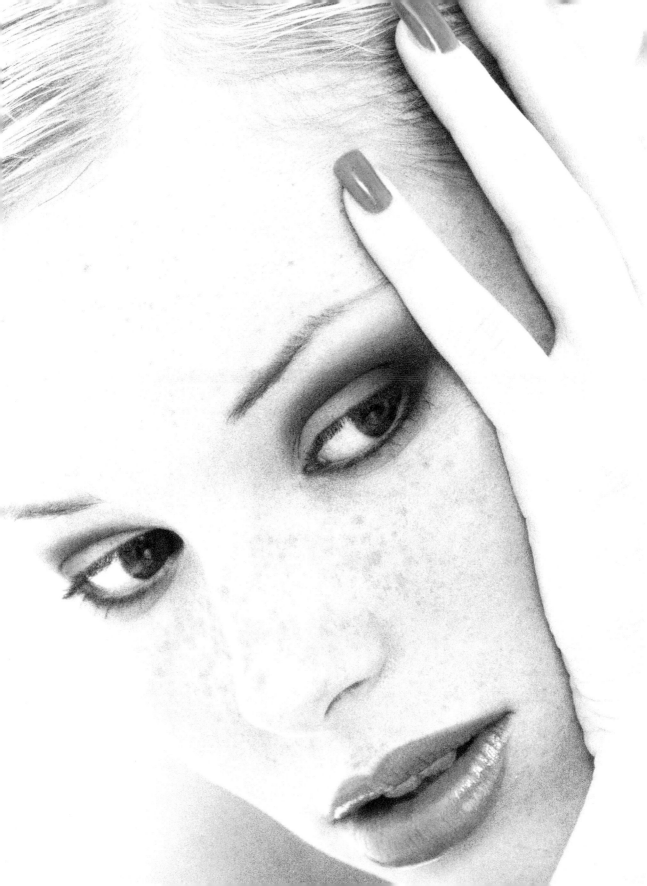

SKIN-CARE REGIMENS

Normal, dry, sensitive, oily, or combination – all skin types need to follow a regular three-stage daily program of cleansing, toning, and moisturizing to keep skin clean, healthy, and in the best condition. But there is no need to stop there. Make the most of the range of special treatments, such as deep-cleansing face masks and gentle scrubs, and take time to enjoy the luxury of a firming facial massage. Here, visual sequences show how to develop the most effective routine for your skin type.

CLEANSING

Cleansing is the first part of your three-stage skin-care regimen and should be done in the morning and again at night to remove both daily grime and deep-down dirt in the pores. Cleansers are also an essential factor in the battle against wrinkles; they help to make skin more receptive to moisturizers and anti-aging treatments. Don't forget to cleanse your neck as well – the skin here needs just as much attention as your face and it is often the first area to show signs of aging.

CHOOSING A CLEANSER

Normal skin	Creamy liquid or cream cleansers; water-soluble cleansers or gentle facial soap.
Dry skin	Cream cleansers or very rich liquid cleansers; moisturizing, nonperfumed soap, but rinse off thoroughly.
Combination or oily skin	Light lotions or milk cleansers; medicated liquid cleansers are sometimes necessary to treat severe outbreaks.
Sensitive skin	Hypoallergenic cleansers; avoid soaps.

1 Keep your hair off your face as much as possible: tie it back or wrap a towel around your head. Make sure that your neck is not covered up with clothing – another reason to cleanse first thing in the morning and last thing at night. To remove eye and lip makeup, see pages 62–63.

2 ◁ Choose a cleanser to suit your skin (see above) and, with your fingertips, massage it all over your face and neck, using small circular movements to work out dirt and other impurities from the skin. Pay particular attention to the T-zone (across the forehead and down the nose to the chin) and the hairline, the areas where most dirt builds up. Always work gently using a soft, light touch rather than a rough abrasive action, which may cause the skin to become red and sore, and can cause long-term damage.

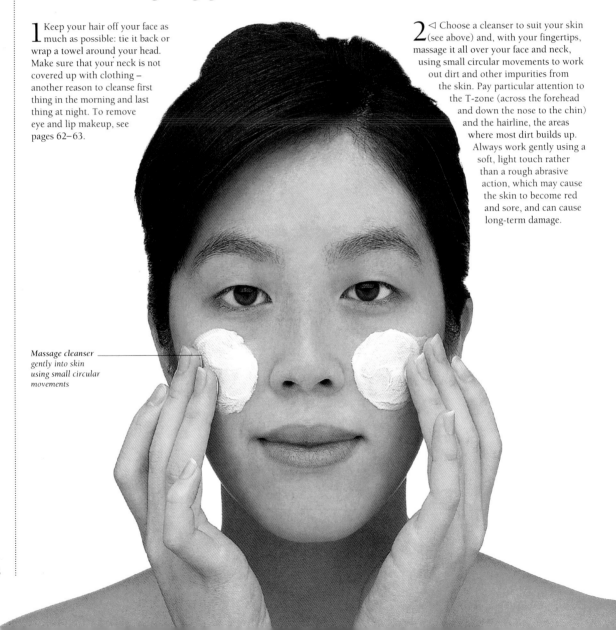

Massage cleanser gently into skin using small circular movements

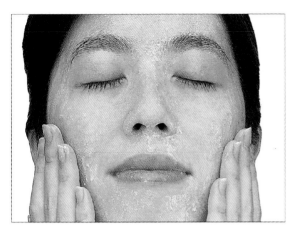

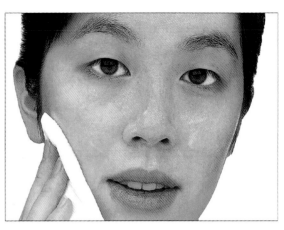

3 If you are using a water-soluble cleanser, rinse your face and neck with water; ideally it should be lukewarm. Warm water helps remove the shine from oily skin, but may irritate dry, sensitive skin; hot water can encourage broken veins.

4 If you are using an oil-soluble cleanser, gently tissue off dirt and grime from the face and neck without dragging or pulling the skin. Change the tissue as soon as it becomes overloaded with dirt; otherwise, you will be working this back into the open pores.

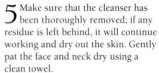

5 Make sure that the cleanser has been thoroughly removed; if any residue is left behind, it will continue working and dry out the skin. Gently pat the face and neck dry using a clean towel.

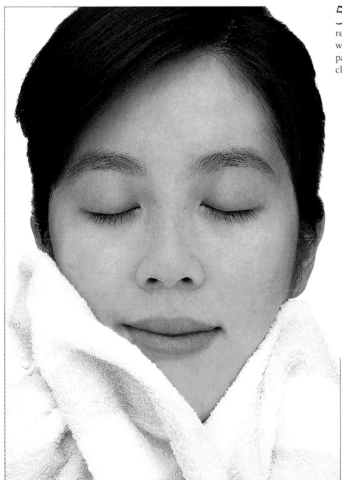

— THE ALLERGY TEST —

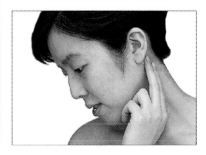

Before buying a cleanser, toner, or moisturizer, test the product. To do this, rub a little behind your ear and check that there is no reaction after 24 hours. If you are choosing products from different makers, test together in the same way.

TONING

Toners, or fresheners, are the second stage in a daily cleansing program. They are designed to remove any last traces of cleanser, while also helping to tighten and refine the pores and prevent a buildup of dead cells. After toning, your skin should feel revitalized and refreshed, and ready to be moisturized. If you think your skin is looking particularly dull, try patting the toner on with a brisk slapping motion, which will stimulate the blood supply to the surface of the skin.

CHOOSING A TONER

Normal skin	*Toners with or without alcohol; rosewater or a still mineral water spray.*
Dry skin	*Mild alcohol-free toners; rosewater or water.*
Combination or oily skin	*Alcohol-based toners (but avoid those with simple alcohols, such as ethanol, methanol, and isopropyl, which can dry the skin).*
Sensitive skin	*Hypoallergenic or alcohol-free toners.*

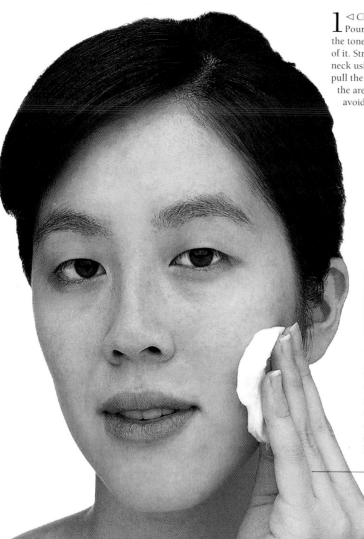

1 ◁ Choose a toner to suit your skin (see above). Pour a little onto a damp cotton ball – this makes the toner easier to apply and also means you use less of it. Stroke the cotton ball gently over your face and neck using small circular movements; do not drag or pull the skin. Concentrate on the T-zone and hairline, the areas where you applied most cleanser, and avoid the delicate eye area and the lips.

2 △ Gently pat your face and neck dry with a clean tissue. If you notice that a toner is beginning to "strip away" your skin, tone with water until the skin becomes rebalanced and then change the product. This often happens with toners that have a very high alcohol content; always check the list of ingredients on the bottle or ask for more information before buying.

Stroke toner gently over the face and neck without dragging the skin

MOISTURIZING

Moisturizers are the final stage in a cleansing program and help restore the moisture loss caused by the drying effects of sunlight, central heating, wind, cold, and pollution. A good daytime moisturizer should contain a sunscreen and will be easily absorbed into the skin. If it leaves an oily film on the surface, it will be difficult to apply makeup on top. At night, you can use a richer, more nourishing cream since this is when your skin most readily absorbs moisture.

CHOOSING A MOISTURIZER

Normal skin	Light creams or lotions, with an added sunscreen.
Dry skin	Protective cream formulas, with an added sunscreen.
Combination or oily skin	Very light, non-oily formulas, with an added sunscreen; should also be noncomedogenic (will not block pores).
Sensitive skin	Hypoallergenic creams, with an added sunscreen.
NIGHT TREATMENT	All skin types should use a richer, more nourishing formula than their daytime moisturizer.

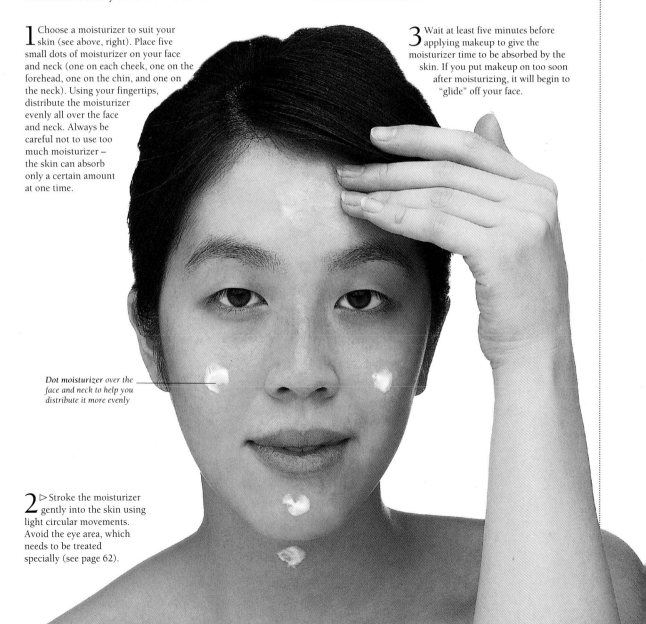

1 Choose a moisturizer to suit your skin (see above, right). Place five small dots of moisturizer on your face and neck (one on each cheek, one on the forehead, one on the chin, and one on the neck). Using your fingertips, distribute the moisturizer evenly all over the face and neck. Always be careful not to use too much moisturizer – the skin can absorb only a certain amount at one time.

3 Wait at least five minutes before applying makeup to give the moisturizer time to be absorbed by the skin. If you put makeup on too soon after moisturizing, it will begin to "glide" off your face.

Dot moisturizer over the face and neck to help you distribute it more evenly

2 ▷ Stroke the moisturizer gently into the skin using light circular movements. Avoid the eye area, which needs to be treated specially (see page 62).

REMOVING EYE MAKEUP

The more eye makeup you wear, the more important it is to use a specially formulated cleanser for the delicate eye area. This makes it much easier to remove even the most stubborn of waterproof or tearproof mascaras without pulling or dragging the sensitive skin around the eyes. If you do not remove all traces of eye makeup whenever you wear it, pores will become blocked, which may lead to pimples. Always use a clean cotton ball, tissue, or cotton swab for each eye.

CARING FOR EYES

◆ Time targets the skin around the eyes first, so it is important to revitalize this area by using an eye cream morning and night.

◆ Use eye creams sparingly; too much can cause puffiness. To apply, place three or four dots below the eye and two on the

brow bone. Stroke the cream in gently using your third, or ring, finger. If you use your index finger, you are more likely to stretch or drag the skin.

◆ Look for ultra-light eye creams with a low oil content as these penetrate the skin more easily.

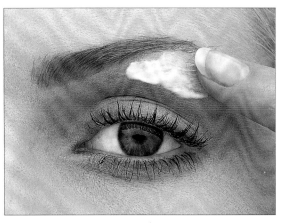

1 To remove makeup from the lids and brows, use the tip of your third finger to stroke in remover gently using small circular movements. Alternatively, use a cotton swab soaked in makeup remover.

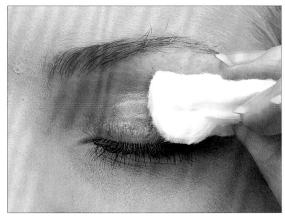

2 Gently wipe off the remover from the lids and brows with a cotton pad, working from the inner corner to the outer corner of the eye. Again, do not rub or drag the skin.

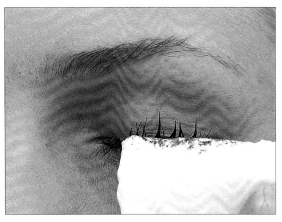

3 To remove mascara, dab a little remover onto a tissue and wrap around your index finger. Brush the tissue through the lashes from underneath.

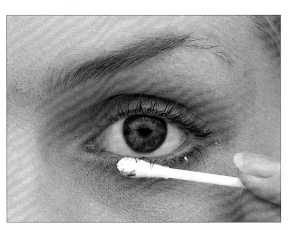

4 For the corner of the eye and the lower lash line, use a cotton swab dipped in remover. Afterward, lightly pat the whole eye area dry with a tissue.

REMOVING LIPSTICK

Always make sure that you remove lipstick thoroughly to prevent the skin on your lips from becoming dry and rough. Lips need to be regularly moisturized, too: they are particularly susceptible to the drying effects of the sun and the wind because they do not have any sebaceous, or oil-producing, glands of their own. If lips are moisturized properly, it is much easier to apply lipstick smoothly and evenly (see pages 96–97), and it will also stay on much better.

CARING FOR LIPS

◆ Use lip moisturizers or lip balms that contain Vitamin E, which is thought to make lips feel extra soft and smooth.

◆ Always use a moisturizing lipstick to prevent lips from drying out during the day and becoming chapped. If you spend a lot of time outdoors, choose lipsticks with a sunscreen.

◆ Combat the appearance of fine wrinkles around the mouth with this simple facial exercise: Open your mouth as wide as you can and resist slightly as you close it. Repeat 10 times.

---

1 Pour a little makeup remover onto a damp cotton ball or tissue and gently wipe in an inward direction, working from each corner to the middle of your lips. Lightly pat dry with a tissue.

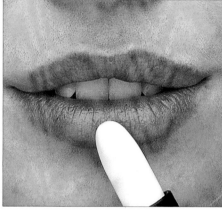

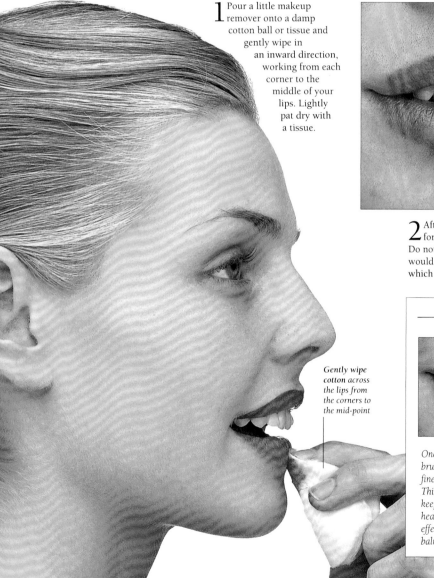

2 After removing lipstick, use a specially formulated lip moisturizer or lip balm. Do not use anything too greasy – that would probably make you lick your lips, which has a drying effect.

Gently wipe cotton across the lips from the corners to the mid-point

---

EXFOLIATING LIPS

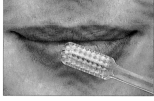

Once a week, exfoliate lips by gently brushing off dead skin with a small, fine brush or a soft toothbrush. This will stimulate cell turnover and keep lips looking smooth, soft, and healthy. For an extra-moisturizing effect, put a little moisturizer or lip balm on the brush.

63

FACE PACKS

Face packs gently remove cells on the skin's surface and purify clogged pores to leave dull skin feeling fresh and firm. They also stimulate blood circulation to give the face a healthy glow and help skin to absorb moisture afterward. Many face packs use natural clay compounds to deep cleanse and remove impurities from the pores. These are perfect for combination and oily skin types, while drier skins should use face packs that are designed to rehydrate or reactivate.

CLEANSING TIPS

◆ *Try to use a face pack about once a week, but never too frequently or the skin will become dry and flaky.*

◆ *If you find it difficult to apply a face pack evenly using your fingertips, try brushing it on with an old makeup brush.*

◆ *When you are waiting for the pack to dry, rest and relax as much as you can (see page 108 for some easy-to-follow relaxation techniques).*

◆ *If possible, wait 24 hours before applying makeup after you have used a face pack.*

COMBINATION SKIN

1 ▷ Cleanse and dry the face thoroughly (see pages 58–59); you should never use face packs on top of makeup as this reduces their cleansing action. Using the fingertips, spread the pack evenly onto the oily areas of the face only, such as the nose and forehead.

2 Wait five to ten minutes for the pack to dry, then rinse off thoroughly with lukewarm water. Massage gently with the fingertips while rinsing to stimulate blood circulation.

3 Pat the face dry with a clean towel and moisturize well (see page 61).

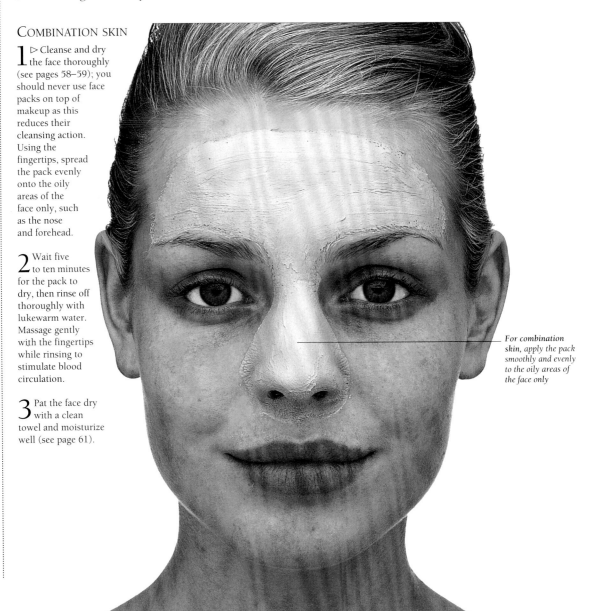

For combination skin, apply the pack smoothly and evenly to the oily areas of the face only

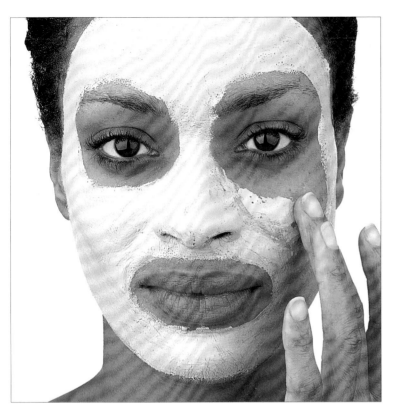

OILY SKIN

1 Cleanse and dry the face thoroughly. Apply the pack evenly, using the fingertips to cover the entire face, but avoid the delicate areas around the eyes and lips. If you are using a rehydrating face pack, follow the same procedure.

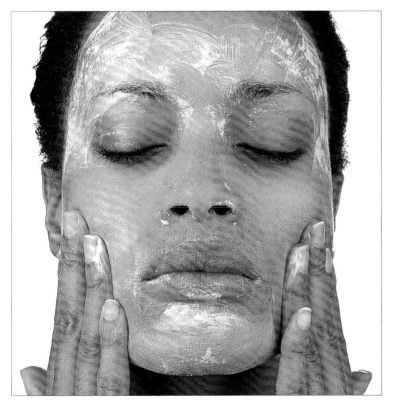

2 ◁ Wait five to ten minutes for the pack to dry completely, then rinse off thoroughly with lukewarm water. Massage gently with the fingertips while rinsing to help remove dull surface cells and to stimulate blood circulation further.

3 Pat the face dry with a clean towel and moisturize well (see page 61).

– BLEMISH TREATMENT–

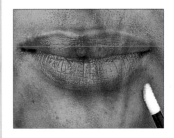

Face packs tend to draw out blemishes. One of the best ways to treat them is with a soft-tipped cleansing stick that can be applied directly to the problem area. This will remove excess oil while also drying out the blemish.

EXFOLIATION

Exfoliation sloughs off dry, dead surface cells to help the skin work more efficiently and look fresher and younger. It also makes skin more receptive to moisturizer and can help keep blemishes at bay. Exfoliate one to three times a week, depending on your skin type – oilier skins should be exfoliated more often, while those with normal and dry skin will find that once a week is sufficient – and preferably at night. Whether a cream or gel, exfoliators should not be abrasive.

CLEANSING TIPS

◆ *Never rub too hard; this not only causes the skin to become sore, but actually stimulates the oil glands to secrete more sebum than before.*

◆ *The first sign of excessive exfoliating is a red and "stripped" look on the delicate skin on the*

upper cheek area. If this happens, stop exfoliating until the skin has recovered completely.

◆ *If you have combination skin, try exfoliating oily areas, such as the T-zone, two to three times a week, and limit yourself to a weekly treatment on dry, sensitive areas.*

1 Cleanse the face (see pages 58–59) and spread exfoliator evenly over it, avoiding the eyes and lips. Let exfoliator dry if necessary.

2 ▷ Rub exfoliator in gently with the fingertips, focusing on any areas of acne. Do not rub too vigorously – if dry patches begin to appear or your skin feels very sensitive, you are probably exfoliating too hard or too often.

3 Rinse your face thoroughly with lukewarm water to remove all traces of exfoliator. Tone and moisturize (see pages 60–61), then wait for a few hours before applying any makeup.

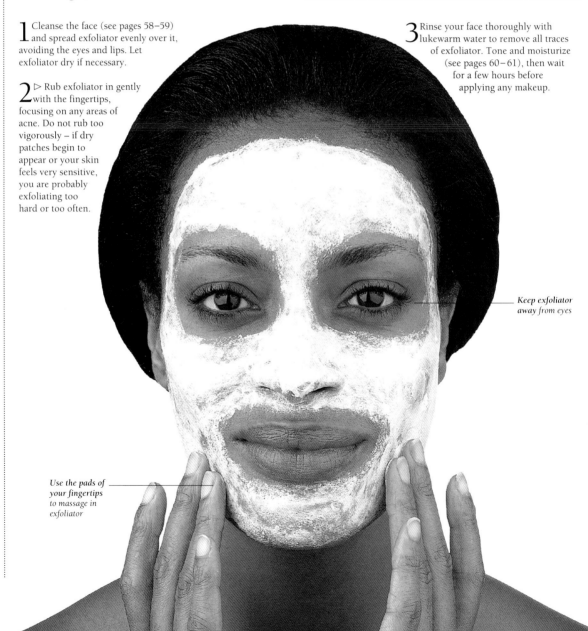

Keep exfoliator
away from eyes

Use the pads of your fingertips to massage in exfoliator

STEAM TOWEL TREATMENT

Hot water is all you need to create your own home sauna. This simple but thorough steaming treatment will help open the pores, loosen blackheads, and draw out pimples, and it will remove deep-down dirt and toxins to leave skin completely clean. It is suitable for all skin types and should be used about once a week as a supplement to your normal cleansing program, although those with very oily skin could use steaming more frequently.

1 Fill a clean bowl three-quarters full with boiling water. Add a few drops of rosewater; it is good for moisturizing the skin.

2 ▷ Position your face about 12–18in (30–45cm) away from the hot water and cover your head and the bowl with a dry towel.

3 Remain in this position for about ten minutes, making sure that the towel still forms a tent around the bowl so that not too much steam escapes.

4 Tone and moisturize the face (see pages 60–61).

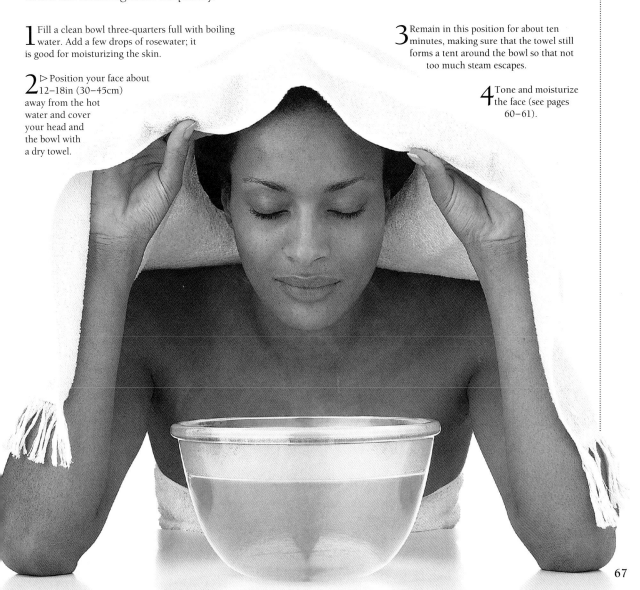

FIRMING FACIAL MASSAGE

Massage has been used throughout the centuries as a way of beautifying and treating the face and body. Although a facial massage will not remove any wrinkles that may already have developed, it can help prevent new lines appearing and make skin look smoother, firmer, and younger. This treatment uses a combination of massage and acupressure techniques to stimulate the flow of blood to the face and encourage the lymph system to drain away any excess fluid, as well as soothing and firming specific points. While massaging, apply a little of your normal face moisturizer or a hot facial massage gel. For maximum benefit, repeat each step about three times and use the middle finger to work on each acupressure point, applying pressure for three seconds at a time and repeating three times. Remember that the skin on the face is more delicate than the rest of your body, so you need to work gently and never use too much pressure or pull the muscles.

FOREHEAD & TEMPLES

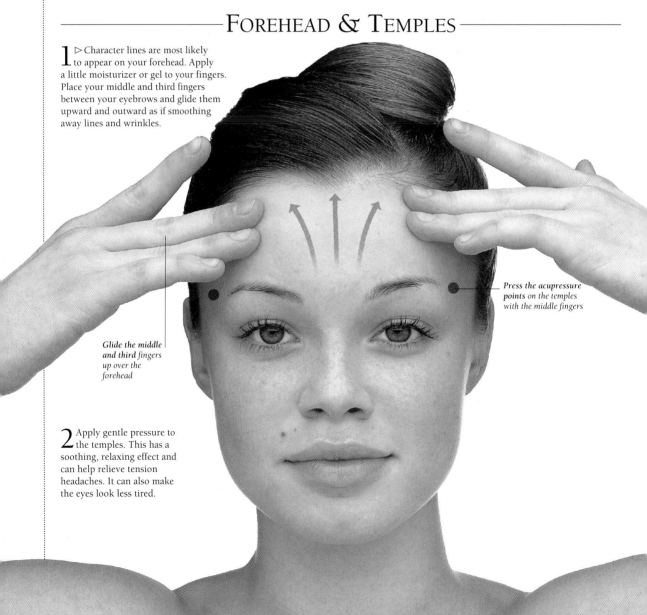

1 ▷ Character lines are most likely to appear on your forehead. Apply a little moisturizer or gel to your fingers. Place your middle and third fingers between your eyebrows and glide them upward and outward as if smoothing away lines and wrinkles.

Press the acupressure points on the temples with the middle fingers

Glide the middle and third fingers up over the forehead

2 Apply gentle pressure to the temples. This has a soothing, relaxing effect and can help relieve tension headaches. It can also make the eyes look less tired.

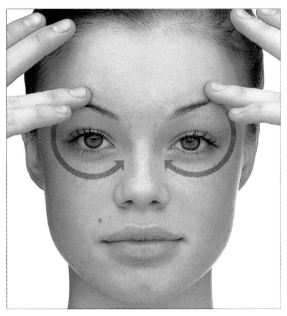

1 To combat the fine lines that easily form around the delicate eye area, circle the third fingers out around the eyes, starting at the inner point of the eyebrows and using a gentle gliding action.

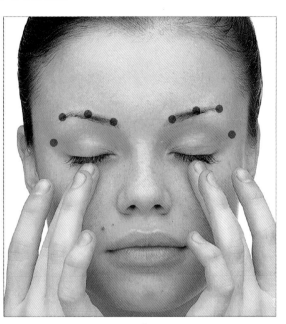

2 Apply pressure to the acupressure points shown along the eyebrows, at the outer corner of the eyes and on the middle point below the eyes. This stimulates blood and lymph flow.

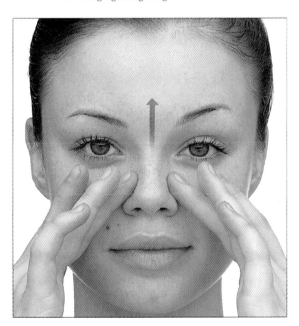

3 Glide your middle finger up along the nose line. Then massage the sides of the nose with the middle fingers in a circular motion to prevent the appearance of fine lines.

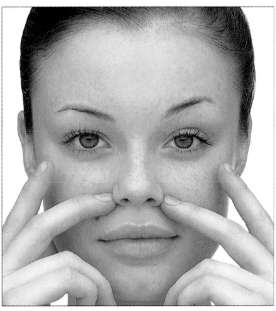

4 Apply pressure to the acupressure points just outside the nostrils. This can help clear a blocked nose and prevent fine lines from appearing around the nose.

CHEEKS & MOUTH

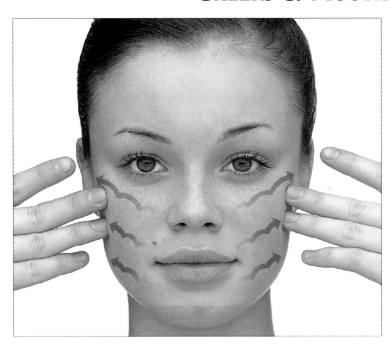

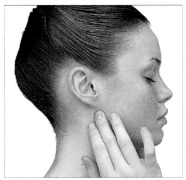

1 ◁ Using the middle and third fingers, massage outward in a spiral motion from the chin to below the earlobes, from the corners of the mouth to the ears and from the sides of the nose to the temples.

2 △ Apply pressure to the acupressure points just below the ears. This stimulates blood and lymph flow to the lower jaw area.

3 ◁ Starting from the center of the chin, use the middle finger to massage around the mouth, working upward to smooth out character lines and wrinkles.

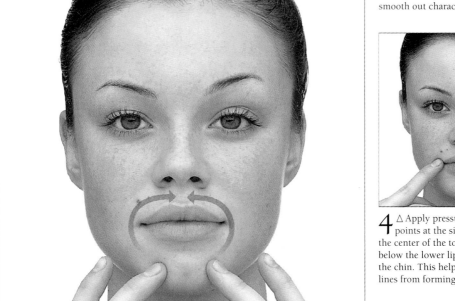

4 △ Apply pressure to the acupressure points at the side of the mouth, above the center of the top lip, the dimple just below the lower lip, and on the center of the chin. This helps prevent character lines from forming around the mouth.

CHIN & NECK

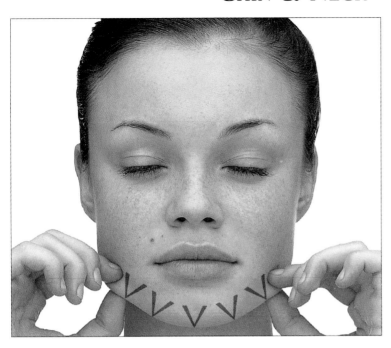

1 ◁ Starting at the edge of the jawbone, use the thumb and forefinger to pinch the skin gently all the way along the jawline to firm up loose flesh. Work toward the center of the chin and back again.

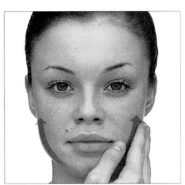

2 △ Glide one palm along the jawline from right to left, then the other palm from left to right. This helps improve tone and reduce sagging along the jawline.

3 ◁ Place your hands at the top of your neck and glide both palms down the neck. This helps stimulate the lymph system into action.

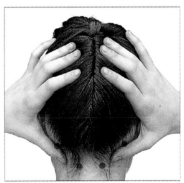

4 △ Apply pressure to the acupressure points shown along the hairline, working from outside the ear to the middle of the neck. This helps reduce tension at the back of the head and neck.

5 Pat lightly all over the face for 30 seconds using your middle three fingers. Rinse off any traces of moisturizer or massage gel with warm water. Pat the face with cold water to tighten pores.

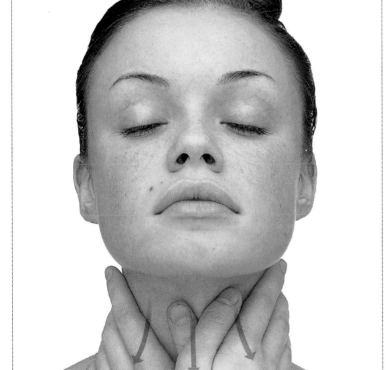

71

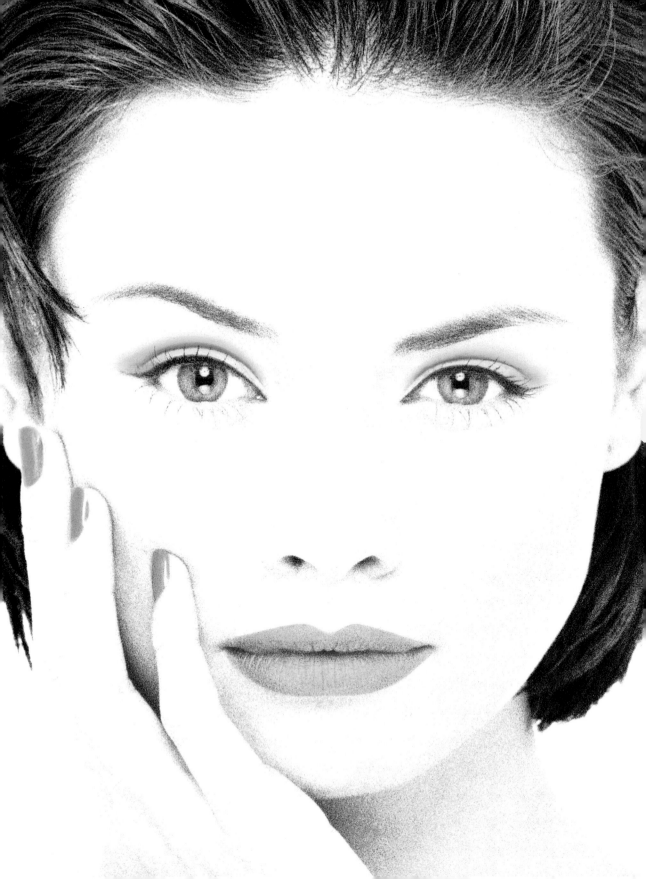

STEP-BY-STEP MAKEUP LESSONS

Applying makeup properly will help you achieve a smooth, professional finish that will last as long as you want it to. Whether you are using eyeshadow or eyeliner, false eyelashes or foundation, lip color or lip liner, there are certain ground rules to follow. The step-by-step photographic makeup lessons on these pages show exactly what you need to do, which equipment to use, and the best way to achieve specific effects for eyes, lips, and nails, as well as how to use color to create different looks.

USING CAKE FOUNDATION

Cake foundations give a smooth, matte finish that prevents skin from looking shiny and oily. Some can be applied using a dry sponge instead of a damp one and many now contain powder particles, with the result that you only need to apply a face powder on top if you have very oily skin. It takes practice to learn how much foundation to use; if you have put too much on, sweep the sponge over the face again but do not reload it.

(see pages 58–61)

PALETTE

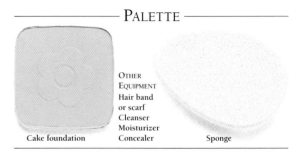

Cake foundation

OTHER
EQUIPMENT
Hair band
or scarf
Cleanser
Moisturizer
Concealer

Sponge

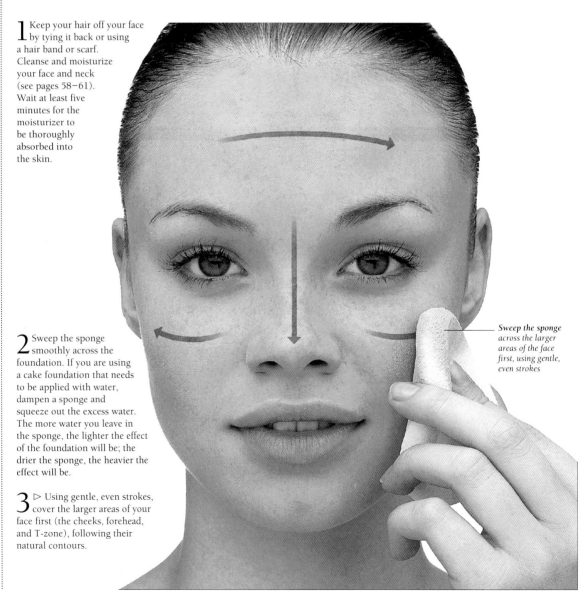

1 Keep your hair off your face by tying it back or using a hair band or scarf. Cleanse and moisturize your face and neck (see pages 58–61). Wait at least five minutes for the moisturizer to be thoroughly absorbed into the skin.

2 Sweep the sponge smoothly across the foundation. If you are using a cake foundation that needs to be applied with water, dampen a sponge and squeeze out the excess water. The more water you leave in the sponge, the lighter the effect of the foundation will be; the drier the sponge, the heavier the effect will be.

3 ▷ Using gentle, even strokes, cover the larger areas of your face first (the cheeks, forehead, and T-zone), following their natural contours.

Sweep the sponge across the larger areas of the face first, using gentle, even strokes

74

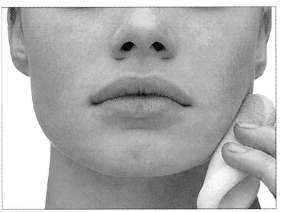

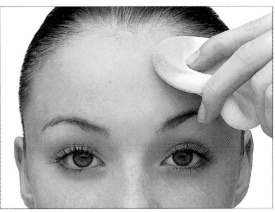

4 Blend well under the jawline and down onto the neck to create a natural effect and avoid a demarcation line.

5 Be careful not to apply too much around the hairline. Finally, check to make sure the face is smoothly and evenly covered. Use a concealer on any blemishes that still show through (see page 77).

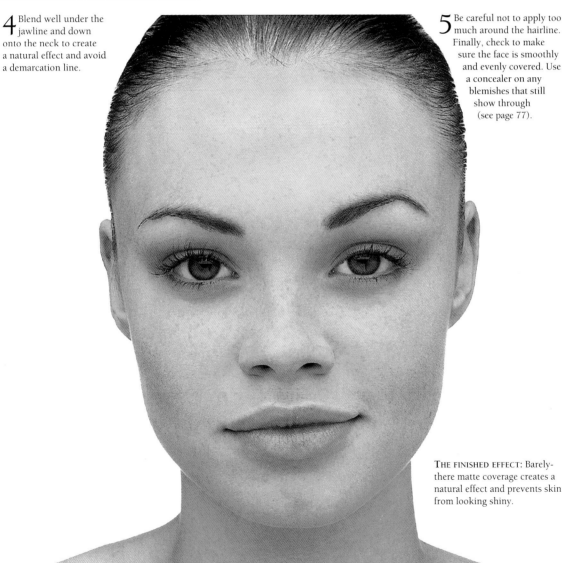

THE FINISHED EFFECT: Barely-there matte coverage creates a natural effect and prevents skin from looking shiny.

USING LIQUID FOUNDATION

Liquid foundation produces a more lightweight finish than the cake variety and tends to be easier to use on dry skin. However, some people find it harder to apply; the trick is not to overload the sponge, which creates a streaky, unnatural effect that will be difficult to correct. To finish, always brush over with a translucent powder. The powder helps the foundation stay in place longer.

PALETTE

Liquid foundation

Translucent powder

Sponge

OTHER EQUIPMENT
Hair band or scarf
Cleanser
Moisturizer
Concealer
and brush
Powder brush

1 Keep your hair off your face by tying it back or using a hair band or scarf. Cleanse your face and neck thoroughly and moisturize (see pages 58–61). Wait at least five minutes for the moisturizer to be thoroughly absorbed into the skin.

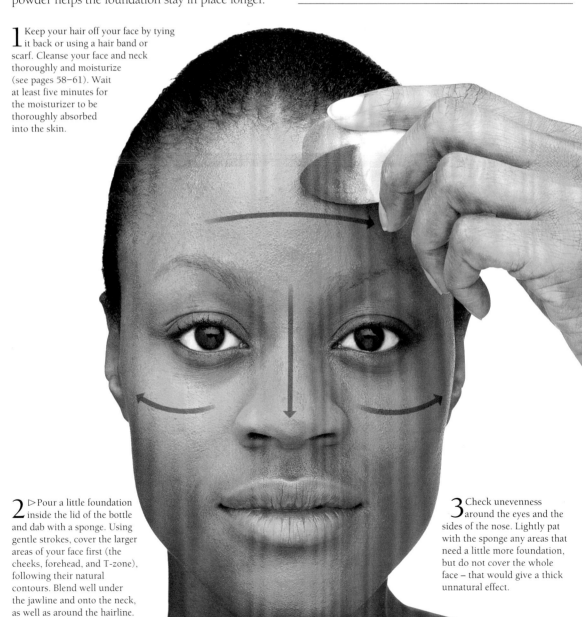

2 ▷ Pour a little foundation inside the lid of the bottle and dab with a sponge. Using gentle strokes, cover the larger areas of your face first (the cheeks, forehead, and T-zone), following their natural contours. Blend well under the jawline and onto the neck, as well as around the hairline.

3 Check unevenness around the eyes and the sides of the nose. Lightly pat with the sponge any areas that need a little more foundation, but do not cover the whole face – that would give a thick unnatural effect.

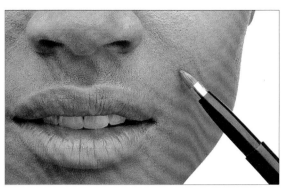

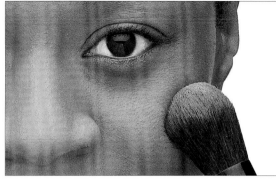

4 If any marks or blemishes still show through, cover them up by brushing on a concealer, blending it well into the surrounding foundation.

5 Brush on a translucent powder, again following the contours of the face. For a more matte effect, apply powder using a soft puff and then brush over.

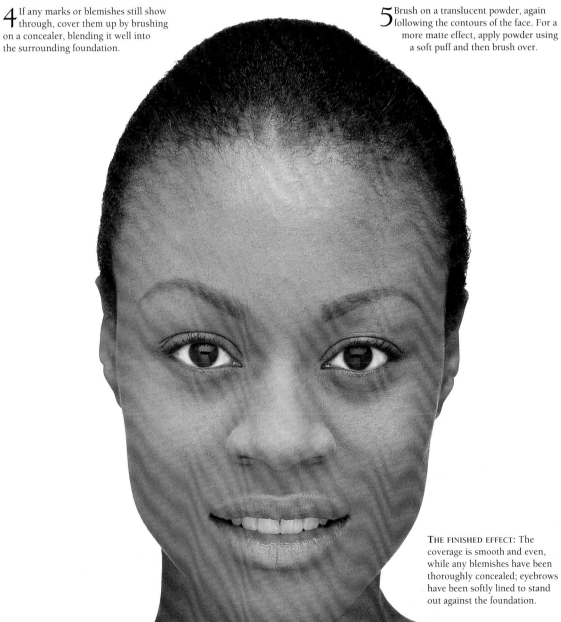

THE FINISHED EFFECT: The coverage is smooth and even, while any blemishes have been thoroughly concealed; eyebrows have been softly lined to stand out against the foundation.

77

COLOR CORRECTING

They may look like the last thing that you would want to put on your face, but liquid color correctors can hide a multitude of sins. They work by using opposing colors to counteract specific flaws in your complexion. For example, green will tone down redness; blue will make a flushed complexion look paler; white will help cover up dark undereye circles and improve dullness; and purple will give a yellowish complexion a healthier glow. Worn underneath foundation, they provide a good base for the rest of your makeup and help it stay fresh longer.

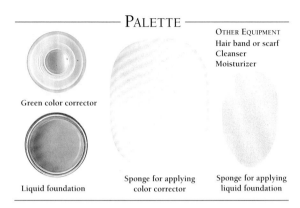

PALETTE

Green color corrector

Liquid foundation

Sponge for applying
color corrector

Sponge for applying
liquid foundation

OTHER EQUIPMENT
Hair band or scarf
Cleanser
Moisturizer

1 Choose the best color corrector for your complexion; green is used here to help counteract redness and broken veins. Keep your hair off your face by tying it back or using a hair band or scarf, and cleanse and moisturize the face and neck (see pages 58–61). Wait about five minutes for the moisturizer to be absorbed.

2 ◁ Pour a little color corrector onto a cosmetic sponge and spread a film of it either all over the face, or just onto specific problem areas such as the cheeks. Check that the coverage is even and reapply the corrector where necessary.

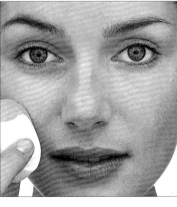

3 Apply liquid foundation as normal (see pages 76–77), making sure that the green does not show through.

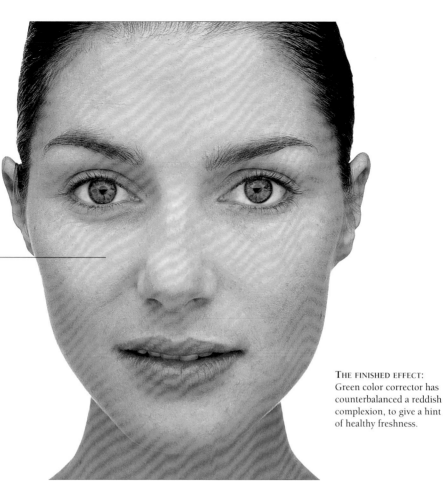

Flushed color and broken veins have been corrected and concealed

THE FINISHED EFFECT: Green color corrector has counterbalanced a reddish complexion, to give a hint of healthy freshness.

CONCEALING UNDEREYE CIRCLES

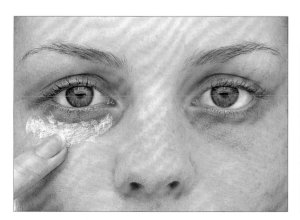

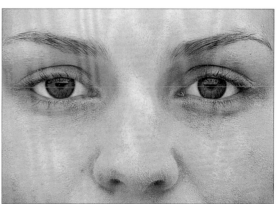

Pour a little white color corrector into one hand and dab some onto your third finger. Smooth fingertip over the dark circle under the eye, making sure the coverage is even.

THE FINISHED EFFECT: Liquid foundation has been applied over the corrector and to the rest of the face, concealing dark undereye circles and giving a smooth finish.

APPLYING BLUSHER

A subtle sweep of blusher will lift your cheekbones and enhance your face. It is applied after foundation, although if you have clear skin you could wear it on its own. Blusher is one of the hardest cosmetics to apply and must be blended perfectly to ensure there are no harsh edges – using a good brush will make it easier. Choose the color carefully: The right shade will make you look healthy, while the wrong one will drain color from your face.

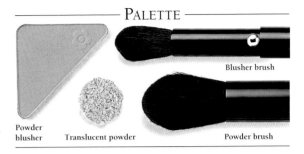

Blusher brush

Powder blusher

Translucent powder

Powder brush

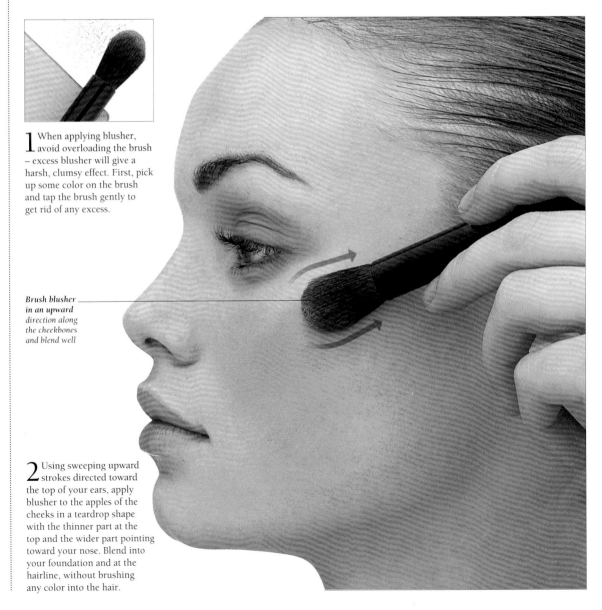

1 When applying blusher, avoid overloading the brush – excess blusher will give a harsh, clumsy effect. First, pick up some color on the brush and tap the brush gently to get rid of any excess.

Brush blusher in an upward direction along the cheekbones and blend well

2 Using sweeping upward strokes directed toward the top of your ears, apply blusher to the apples of the cheeks in a teardrop shape with the thinner part at the top and the wider part pointing toward your nose. Blend into your foundation and at the hairline, without brushing any color into the hair.

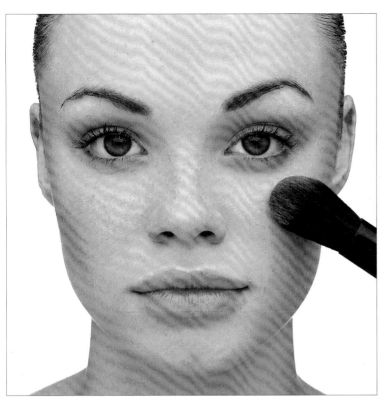

3 If you think you have put on too much blusher, brush over with a little translucent powder (see page 77) to tone down the color. Once you have finished the rest of your makeup, check that you have applied enough blusher and, if necessary, add a little more.

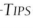

TIPS

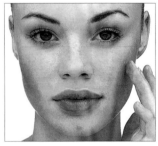

◆ *For a slightly more girlish look using either powder or cream blusher, apply circles of blusher on the apples of your cheeks (see above) and blend well.*

◆ *Cream blusher, which glides on easily, can be used to create a more natural look and works well with liquid foundation. Pick up some color on your fingertips and apply to the cheeks in a teardrop shape. Blend in using a gentle circular motion.*

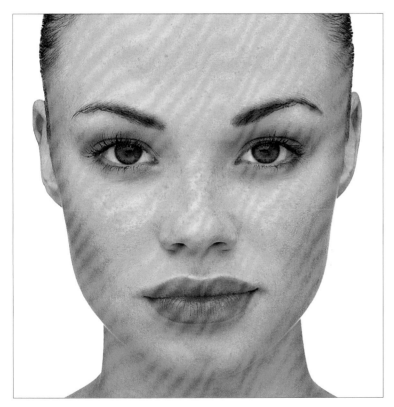

THE FINISHED EFFECT: Blusher has been used to enhance the shape of the face and lift the cheekbones, while lips have been lightly brushed with a related shade.

SHADING & HIGHLIGHTING

Whatever shape your face, skillful shading and highlighting can help to enhance your good points and minimize the less desirable ones. Using a lighter shade of foundation than your overall base, highlighting makes features more prominent, while shading uses a darker tone to make features recede into the background. You should highlight good points, such as high cheekbones, but shadow plump cheeks or a heavy jawline.

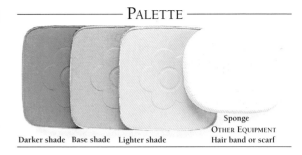

PALETTE

Darker shade   Base shade   Lighter shade

Sponge
OTHER EQUIPMENT
Hair band or scarf

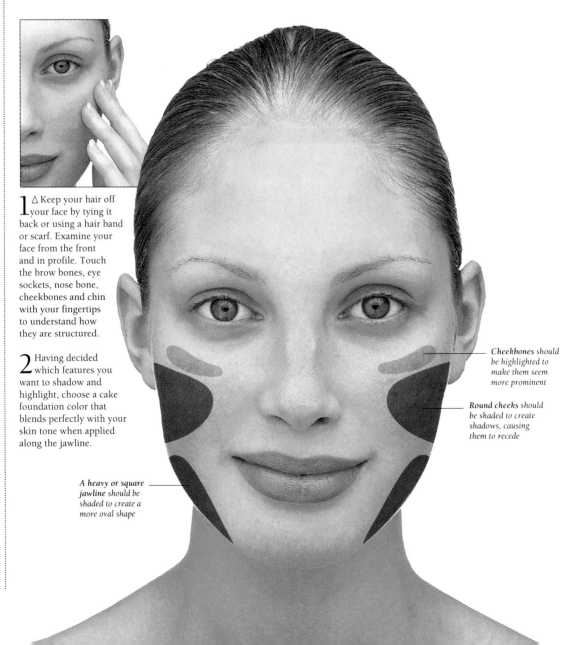

1 △ Keep your hair off your face by tying it back or using a hair band or scarf. Examine your face from the front and in profile. Touch the brow bones, eye sockets, nose bone, cheekbones and chin with your fingertips to understand how they are structured.

2 Having decided which features you want to shadow and highlight, choose a cake foundation color that blends perfectly with your skin tone when applied along the jawline.

Cheekbones should be highlighted to make them seem more prominent

Round cheeks should be shaded to create shadows, causing them to recede

A heavy or square jawline should be shaded to create a more oval shape

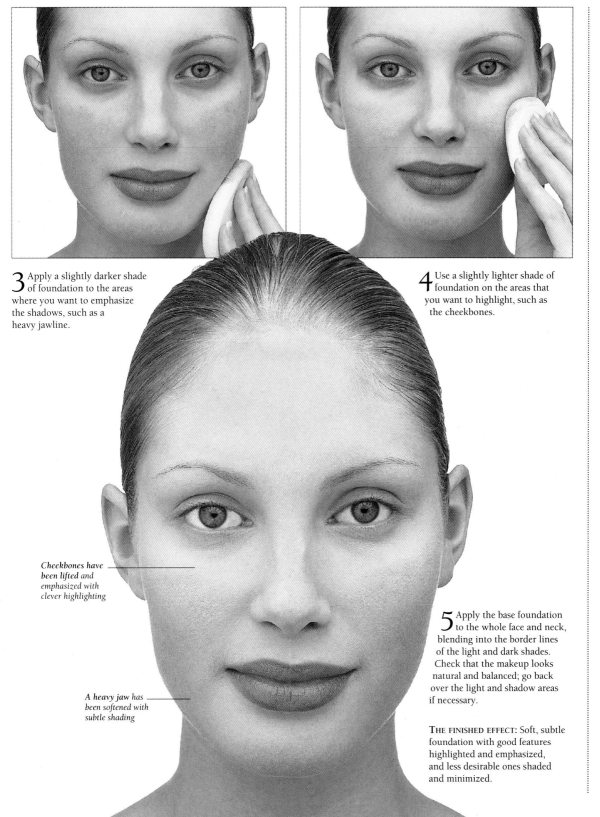

3 Apply a slightly darker shade of foundation to the areas where you want to emphasize the shadows, such as a heavy jawline.

4 Use a slightly lighter shade of foundation on the areas that you want to highlight, such as the cheekbones.

Cheekbones have been lifted and emphasized with clever highlighting

A heavy jaw has been softened with subtle shading

5 Apply the base foundation to the whole face and neck, blending into the border lines of the light and dark shades. Check that the makeup looks natural and balanced; go back over the light and shadow areas if necessary.

THE FINISHED EFFECT: Soft, subtle foundation with good features highlighted and emphasized, and less desirable ones shaded and minimized.

83

CORRECTING FACE SHAPES

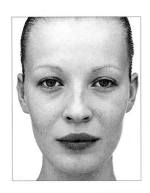

LONG To reduce the length of a long face, use a darker shade of foundation to shade around the top of the forehead, blending it into the hairline. Shade along the jawline, too, and under the cheekbones. Dot a lighter shade just above the cheekbones to highlight, then apply the base foundation, blending well. Reapply the lighter and darker shades if necessary. Brush blusher along the cheekbones but not too far down the face.

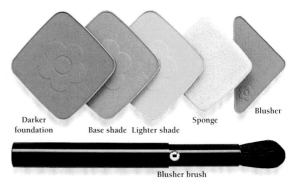

Darker foundation   Base shade   Lighter shade   Sponge   Blusher

Blusher brush

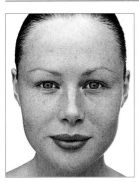

SQUARE Soften a square face by using a darker foundation to shade an almost triangular shape on either side of the jaw. Shade the sides of the forehead, too, to help reduce the width of the top part of the face. Dot a lighter shade above the cheekbones to highlight, then apply base foundation, blending well. Reapply the lighter and darker shades if necessary. Brush blusher along the cheekbones.

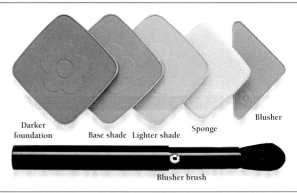

Darker foundation   Base shade   Lighter shade   Sponge   Blusher

Blusher brush

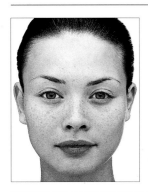

ROUND To reduce the width of a round face, use a darker foundation underneath the cheekbones to give the face more angles. Blend up into the hairline. Dot a lighter shade above the cheekbones to highlight and on the tip of the chin to counteract the moon shape. Apply the base foundation and blend well. Reapply the lighter and darker shades if necessary. Brush blusher along the cheekbones.

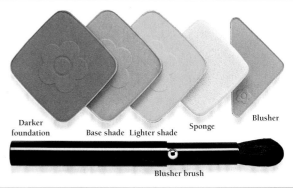

Darker foundation   Base shade   Lighter shade   Sponge   Blusher

Blusher brush

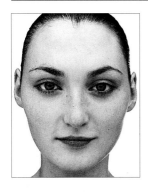

HEART To even up a heart-shaped face, use a darker shade of foundation on the sides of the forehead to help reduce the width of the face, and also on the tip of the chin to make it look less pointed. Dot a lighter shade just above the cheekbones to highlight, then apply the base foundation, blending well. Reapply the lighter and darker shades if necessary. Brush blusher along the cheekbones blending it up onto the temples.

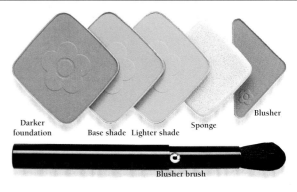

Darker foundation   Base shade   Lighter shade   Sponge   Blusher

Blusher brush

ACHIEVING THE EFFECT———THE FINAL LOOK

Shade around top of the forehead

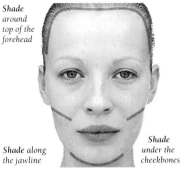

Shade along the jawline

Shade under the cheekbones

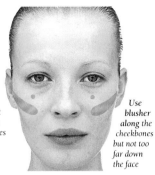

Highlight above the cheekbones

Use blusher along the cheekbones but not too far down the face

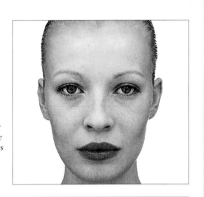

Shade the sides of the forehead

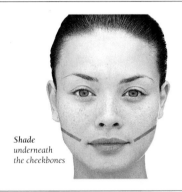

Shade on both sides of the jaw

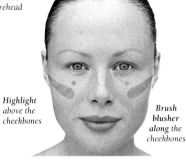

Highlight above the cheekbones

Brush blusher along the cheekbones

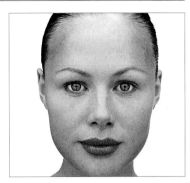

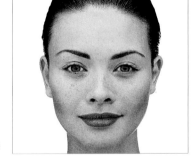

Shade underneath the cheekbones

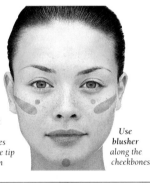

Highlight above the cheekbones and on the tip of the chin

Use blusher along the cheekbones

Shade sides of the forehead

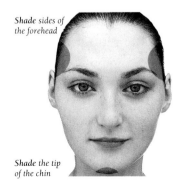

Shade the tip of the chin

Highlight above the cheekbones

Blend blusher along the cheekbones and onto the temples

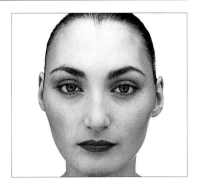

85

APPLYING EYESHADOW

Dark and dramatic, light and pearly, frosted and fresh – a wide variety of effects can be achieved with eyeshadows (see A Gallery of Looks, pages 8–25). However, the general rule is to use four different-colored shadows; a neutral-toned base, a main color, a darker shade for emphasizing, and a lighter shade for highlighting. It is also important to use a magnifying mirror so you can see exactly what you are doing, and to keep a good range of different-sized brushes, or sponge-tipped applicators, to hand to help you blend the shadows well and prevent harsh lines.

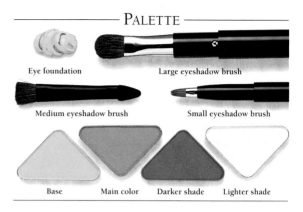

PALETTE

Eye foundation

Large eyeshadow brush

Medium eyeshadow brush

Small eyeshadow brush

Base · Main color · Darker shade · Lighter shade

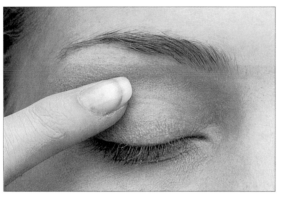

1 Cover the whole eye area with a specially formulated eye foundation, working from the top lash line to the eyebrow. Gently rub the foundation into the skin with your fingertip and allow to dry.

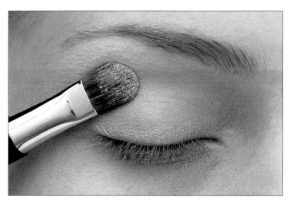

2 With a large eyeshadow brush, apply the neutral-colored base eyeshadow all over the eye area, working from the eyelashes to the eyebrow and blending out very slightly at the corner.

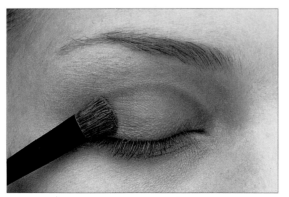

3 With a medium brush, apply the main color eyeshadow to the eyelid up to the socket line. Start from the inside corner and work outward, but avoid building up color at the inner corner.

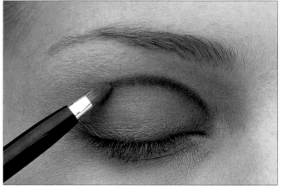

4 Use a small, more pointed eyeshadow brush to run the slightly darker shade of the main color in a thin line along the socket line, working from the inside corner outward.

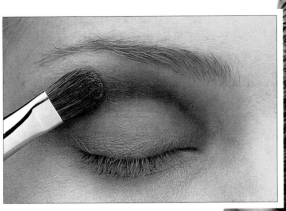

5 For a dramatic effect, leave the line along the socket. For a softer look, blend it in well using the large brush, or a cotton swab.

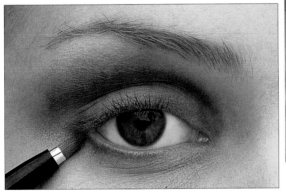

6 Using the small brush, apply the darker color in a line underneath the bottom lashes, starting about halfway along the eye and working to the outer corner.

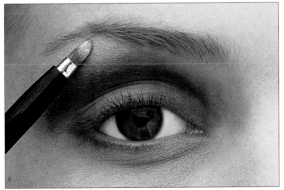

7 Run the small brush against the back of your hand to remove color. Then use it to apply the lighter, pearlier shade just under the brow area. Be careful not to apply any color to the eyebrows.

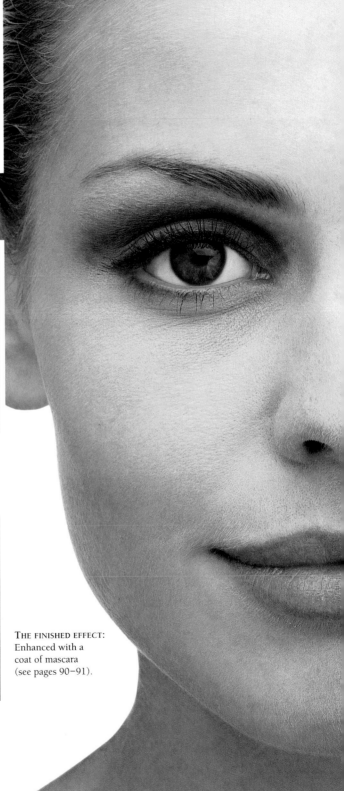

THE FINISHED EFFECT: Enhanced with a coat of mascara (see pages 90–91).

APPLYING LIQUID EYELINER

Liquid eyeliner is the hardest eye definer to apply. It demands the steadiest hand, but it does give the most effective finish. It can be put on before or after eyeshadow, but if you apply it before it is easier to cover up any mistakes that you might make. Always start by blotting the liner brush on a tissue to make sure it is not overloaded.

── PALETTE ──

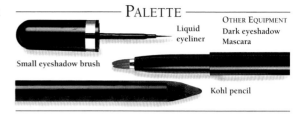

Liquid eyeliner

OTHER EQUIPMENT
Dark eyeshadow
Mascara

Small eyeshadow brush

Kohl pencil

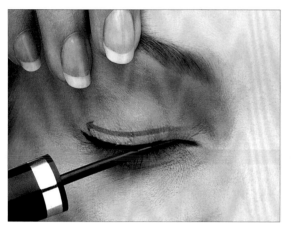

1 Holding the skin slightly taut, position the liner brush at the inner corner of your eye, resting on the top lashes. Sweep along the upper lash line to the outer corner, drawing outward. Let dry for 10 seconds and go back over the line again.

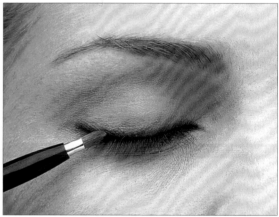

2 For a striking effect, leave the eyeliner as it is. For a softer look, brush over it with a little dark eyeshadow using a small, pointed eyeshadow brush, but be careful not to press hard and smudge the eyeliner too much.

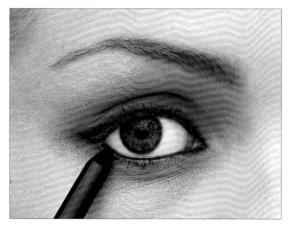

3 It is generally better not to line the lower lashes with liquid eyeliner; this creates a very harsh effect. Either use an eyeshadow (see page 87) or run a kohl pencil along the inner rim of the eye, taking it right into the inner corner.

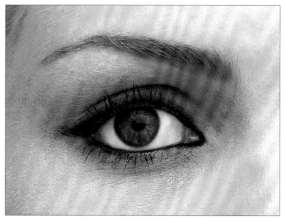

THE FINISHED EFFECT: The top lash line has been smoothly outlined with liquid eyeliner, while black kohl pencil applied along the bottom inner rim of the eye creates a smoky, sultry effect. A light coat of mascara adds the perfect finishing touch.

APPLYING FALSE EYELASHES

For special occasions when you want to create a dramatic effect, try enhancing and lengthening your top lashes with false eyelashes. These should be applied after eyeshadow and eyeliner, and are not as hard to put on as you might think. To remove, hold the outside edge of the lash and peel off as gently but as quickly as you can.

PALETTE

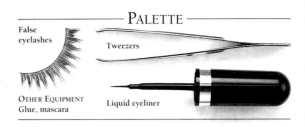

False eyelashes

Tweezers

OTHER EQUIPMENT
Glue, mascara

Liquid eyeliner

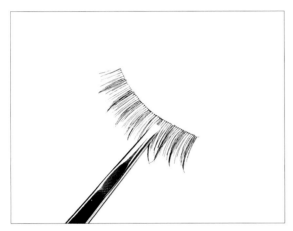

1 Pick up a false eyelash with a pair of clean tweezers and, using your other hand, run a small amount of glue (normally supplied with a set of false eyelashes) along the top edge. Wait about 30 seconds for the glue to dry slightly.

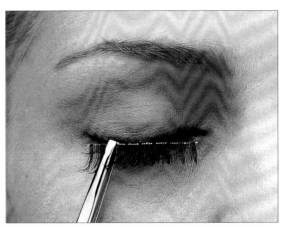

2 Line up the outer edge of the false eyelash against the outer edge of your own lashes. Push as close as possible into the roots and try not to panic. Make sure the eyelash is secure at both corners as well as at the center of the lid.

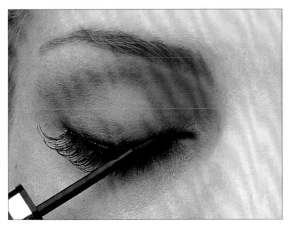

3 Keep the eye closed for 30 seconds and then run a thin line of liquid eyeliner over the "seam" to give a neat finish.

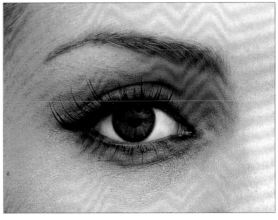

THE FINISHED EFFECT: False eyelashes lengthened with a little mascara give the eye a dramatic, glamorous look.

APPLYING MASCARA

How many coats you apply and whether or not you use mascara on the bottom lashes really depends on the style of makeup you want to achieve (see A Gallery of Looks, pages 8–25). But if you are applying more than one coat, allow the first to dry before starting the second. Always take mascara into the inner corners of the top lashes, which helps to make eyes look larger.

── PALETTE ──

Eyelash comb or old
mascara wand

OTHER EQUIPMENT
Eyelash curler
Tissue
Magnifying mirror
Cotton swab
Eye makeup remover

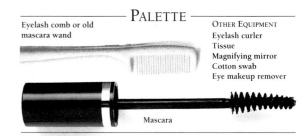

Mascara

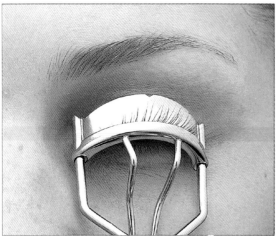

1 If your eyelashes are particularly straight, curl them with an eyelash curler. This will immediately open up the eyes and make them look bigger. But do not press too hard – it could create a kink in the middle of the lashes – and remember to open up the curlers fully before pulling them away from your eye.

2 If you want to apply mascara to the bottom lashes, do so before coating the top lashes. It is very important not to put too much mascara on the bottom lashes, so make sure the wand is not overloaded by wiping off any excess on a tissue.

3 ▷Hold a magnifying mirror slightly above your face and position the wand vertically straight in front of you. Stroke down the bottom lashes, working from the inner to the outer corner of the eye.

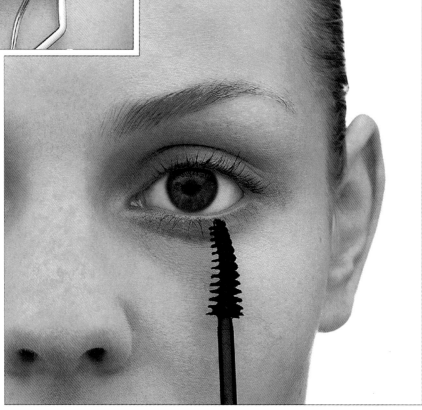

90

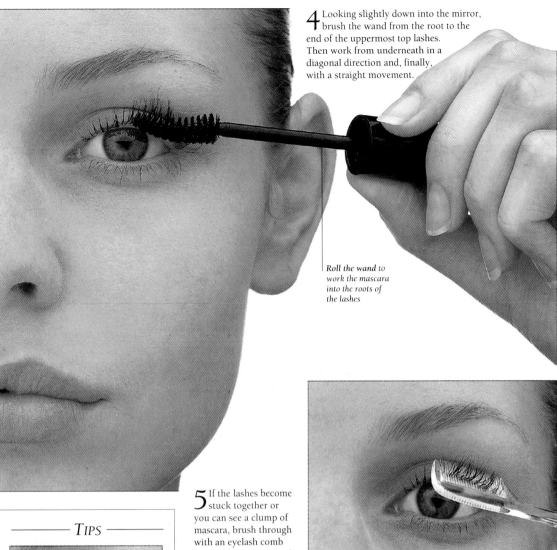

4 Looking slightly down into the mirror, brush the wand from the root to the end of the uppermost top lashes. Then work from underneath in a diagonal direction and, finally, with a straight movement.

Roll the wand to work the mascara into the roots of the lashes

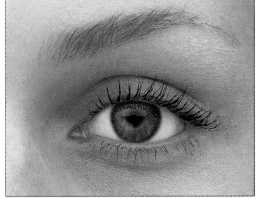

5 If the lashes become stuck together or you can see a clump of mascara, brush through with an eyelash comb or an old mascara wand.

TIPS

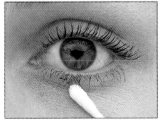

◆ *In case of smudges, dip a cotton swab into some non-oily eye makeup remover and gently rub off unwanted mascara as shown above.*

◆ *To prevent a mascara wand from becoming too clogged, wash through with soapy water, rinse, and let dry completely before using.*

THE FINISHED EFFECT: The eye has been opened up and defined by applying mascara to the top and bottom lashes.

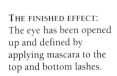

91

DEFINING EYEBROWS

Well-groomed eyebrows help draw attention to the eyes and make them look bigger. Eyebrow fashions change frequently, so the most sensible option is to stick to a natural but cared-for look, unless you deliberately want to create a more dramatic and defined effect. Eyebrow color should relate to your hair color and the overall strength of the makeup you are using. It is often better to choose a shade that is slightly lighter than the color you first thought of.

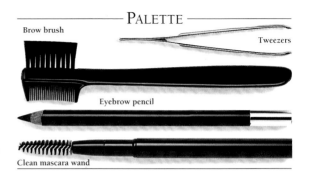

PALETTE

Brow brush

Tweezers

Eyebrow pencil

Clean mascara wand

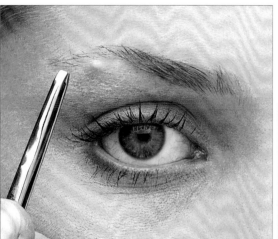

1 If necessary, pluck away any loose, straggly hairs with a pair of tweezers. Always pluck from underneath the brow and pull hairs in the direction they are growing using a swift, sharp movement. Pluck one hair at a time, and remember it is better to pluck too few than too many.

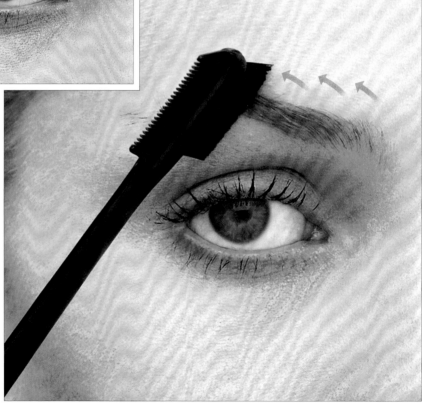

2 Brush eyebrows into shape using a brow brush. Work upward and outward to give the brow more definition and help open up the whole eye area.

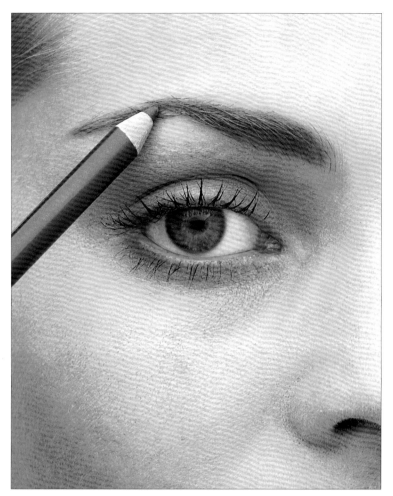

3 ◁ With an eyebrow pencil, use light, feathery strokes to fill in any gaps in your eyebrows. Extend the eyebrow very slightly at the outer corner and accentuate the natural arch of the brow.

4 Brush through again with the brow brush to blend in the eyebrow pencil, again working upward and outward.

---*TIPS*---

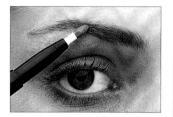

◆ *For a softer, more natural look, you can use an eyeshadow rather than an eyebrow pencil. Apply using a small, pointed brush and then brush through.*

◆ *For Audrey Hepburn-style eyebrows, brush brows upward more vigorously and then soften with eyeshadow.*

◆ *The best time to pluck your eyebrows is after a bath or shower; then the hairs will come out much more easily.*

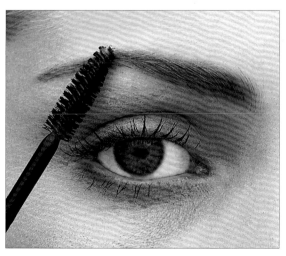

5 To keep individual hairs in place, spray a little hairspray onto an old, clean mascara wand and comb gently through the eyebrow.

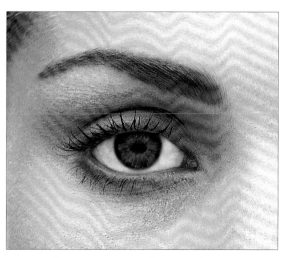

THE FINISHED EFFECT: The natural shape and arch of the eyebrow has been gently emphasized to help frame and accentuate the whole eye area.

93

EFFECTS FOR EYES

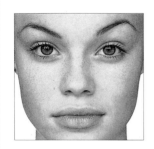

DEEP-SET EYES Enhance deeper eyes by shaping the brows and softening with a brown pencil. Apply a gold shadow over the eye area and a rust shadow along the socket line. Blend well. Line the top and bottom lash lines with a reddish brown shadow. Brush to soften. Lightly coat the top lashes with black mascara.

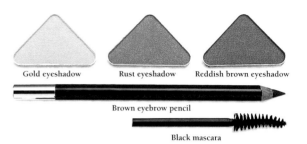

Gold eyeshadow   Rust eyeshadow   Reddish brown eyeshadow

Brown eyebrow pencil

Black mascara

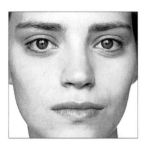

HEAVY BROWS To balance heavy brows, brush into shape, then apply a lilac shadow over the eye area. Dot a white shadow at the inner corner. Use a violet shadow at the outer corner and on the lower lash line. Use black kohl on the bottom rim and black liquid liner on the top lash line. Coat the lashes with black mascara.

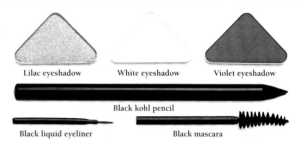

Lilac eyeshadow   White eyeshadow   Violet eyeshadow

Black kohl pencil

Black liquid eyeliner   Black mascara

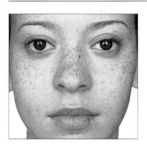

ROUND EYES Highlight round eyes by softening brows with a brown pencil. Apply a pale green shadow over the eye area and under the lower lash line, and add a dark green to the lid. Smudge a charcoal shadow along the top lash line and line with black liquid liner, drawing outward. Sweep black mascara through the top lashes.

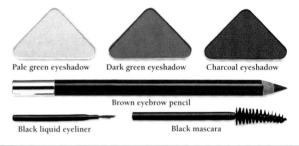

Pale green eyeshadow   Dark green eyeshadow   Charcoal eyeshadow

Brown eyebrow pencil

Black liquid eyeliner   Black mascara

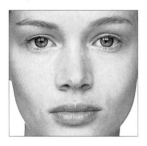

SMALL EYES Enlarge smaller eyes by shaping brows with a brown pencil and using a pale pink shadow over the eye area. Circle the eye with a brown shadow, smudging underneath. Apply soft black shadow to the lid. Line the top lash line with black liquid liner, brushing over with black shadow. Coat the lashes with black mascara.

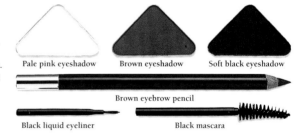

Pale pink eyeshadow   Brown eyeshadow   Soft black eyeshadow

Brown eyebrow pencil

Black liquid eyeliner   Black mascara

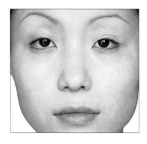

ASIAN EYES To define Asian eyes, softly arch the brows and fill any gaps with a gray pencil. Apply a white shadow over the eye area. Softly line the socket with a gray shadow and run a thin line of blue shadow along the top and bottom lash lines, drawing out at the corner. Coat the top and bottom lashes with cobalt blue mascara.

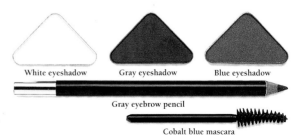

White eyeshadow   Gray eyeshadow   Blue eyeshadow

Gray eyebrow pencil

Cobalt blue mascara

ACHIEVING THE LOOK ——————— THE FINAL LOOK

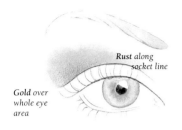

Gold over whole eye area

Rust along socket line

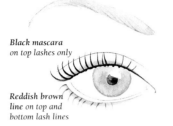

Black mascara on top lashes only

Reddish brown line on top and bottom lash lines

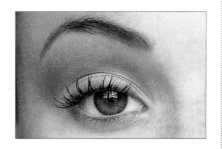

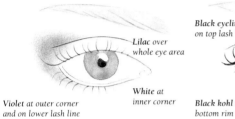

Lilac over whole eye area

Violet at outer corner and on lower lash line

White at inner corner

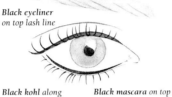

Black eyeliner on top lash line

Black kohl along bottom rim

Black mascara on top and bottom lashes

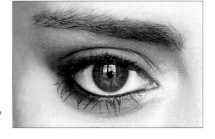

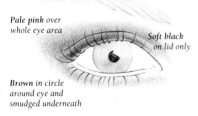

Pale green over whole eye area and under lower lash line

Dark green on lid only

Charcoal on top lash line

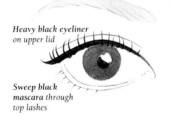

Heavy black eyeliner on upper lid

Sweep black mascara through top lashes

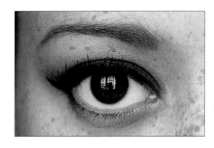

Pale pink over whole eye area

Soft black on lid only

Brown in circle around eye and smudged underneath

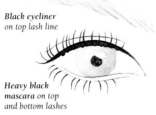

Black eyeliner on top lash line

Heavy black mascara on top and bottom lashes

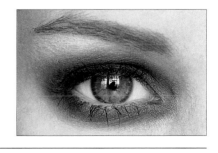

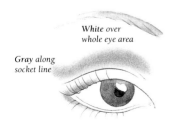

White over whole eye area

Gray along socket line

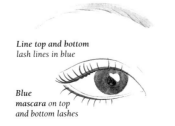

Line top and bottom lash lines in blue

Blue mascara on top and bottom lashes

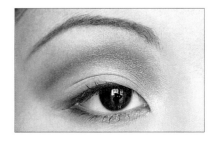

APPLYING LIPSTICK & LIP LINER

Lipstick adds the finishing touch to makeup. It should help unite the other colors you have used and really bring your face alive. However, if it is badly applied, it will look clumsy and unsubtle. The answer is to use a lip liner to give lips a neat, defined edge and to build up color using a lip brush. To make the most of your individual lip shape, or to correct a particular problem, see Effects for Lips (pages 98–99).

PALETTE

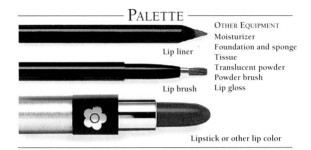

Lip liner

Lip brush

Lipstick or other lip color

OTHER EQUIPMENT
Moisturizer
Foundation and sponge
Tissue
Translucent powder
Powder brush
Lip gloss

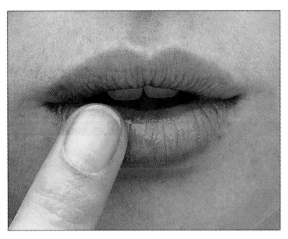

1 Soften lips by gently rubbing on a small amount of moisturizer. This will help the lipstick to glide on more easily.

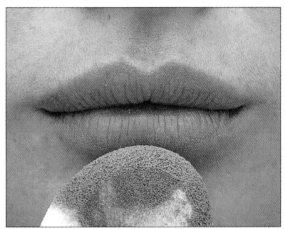

2 Apply a very light touch of your normal foundation to act as a base and help even out the color.

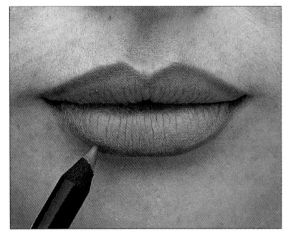

3 Outline the natural edge of the lips with a lip liner that is not more than one shade darker than your chosen lip color. This keeps color from bleeding and gives a guideline for applying lipstick.

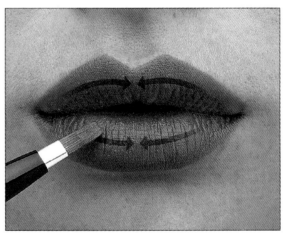

4 Use a lip brush to apply lipstick; this gives you more control over direction. Relax your mouth so that it falls slightly open and brush on color from the corners to the middle point of both lips.

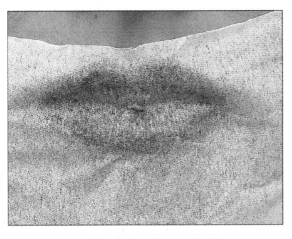

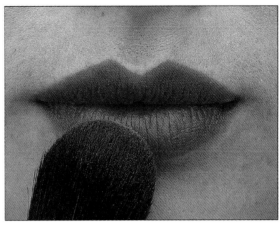

5 Press lips gently with a tissue, but be careful not to smudge the color or to remove too much. Then brush on more color to create a deeper effect.

6 For a matte effect, dust lips lightly with translucent powder using a powder brush. For a shiny finish, use a clear or colored lip gloss on top of lipstick.

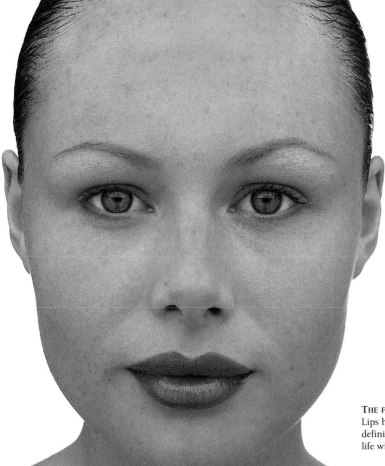

TIPS

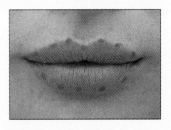

◆ *If you find it hard to keep your hand steady while applying lip liner, try placing dots at strategic points around your lips and then connecting them. Be careful not to make the dots too large.*

◆ *To prevent lipstick from sticking to your teeth, put a finger inside your mouth and draw out slowly to remove any excess from the inside of the lips.*

◆ *Lip liners are easier to sharpen if you put them in the refrigerator for about 30 minutes beforehand.*

THE FINISHED EFFECT:
Lips have been given extra definition and brought to life with a burst of color.

EFFECTS FOR LIPS

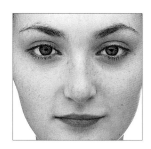

THIN LIPS Make thin lips look fuller and accentuate their shape by outlining just outside their natural edge with a lip liner. Brush on a lip color inside the line you have drawn. Avoid using very matte colors as these can make lips look even thinner; slightly glossy colors will make lips look fuller.

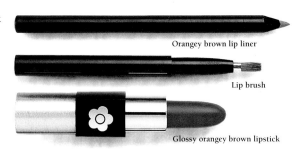

Orangey brown lip liner

Lip brush

Glossy orangey brown lipstick

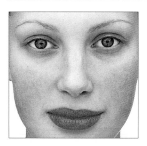

UNEVEN LIPS Balance an uneven top lip by outlining just outside the thinner half of the lip and along the natural edge of the fuller half using a lip liner. Check that the line is even, then outline the lower lip. Brush on a lip color inside the line. If lips still look uneven, add more color to the thinner half of the lip.

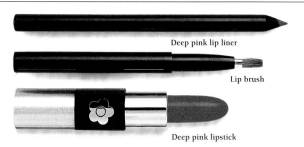

Deep pink lip liner

Lip brush

Deep pink lipstick

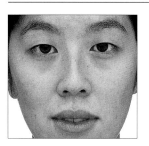

SHAPELESS LIPS Give lips more definition by outlining the top lip with a lip liner to emphasize the "m" in the middle and so create more of a cupid's bow. Outline just outside the natural edge of the lower lip to make it look fuller. Brush on a strong lip color to help give the lips even more definition.

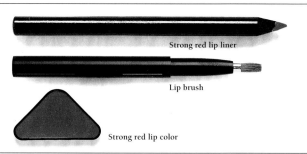

Strong red lip liner

Lip brush

Strong red lip color

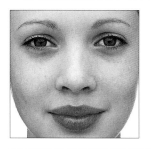

FULL LIPS Make full lips appear thinner by lightly covering them with foundation to help blur the edges. Using a lip liner, outline lips just inside their natural edge, then brush on a lip color, being careful not to go outside the line. Avoid pearly or glossy colors as these will make the lips look even fuller.

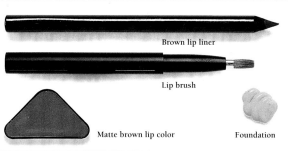

Brown lip liner

Lip brush

Matte brown lip color

Foundation

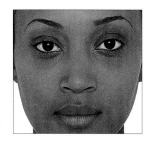

UNEVEN COLOR Balance different-colored lips by covering both with a little foundation. Outline lips with a lip liner, then brush a darker shade of your chosen lip color onto the lip that looks lighter and a lighter shade onto the one that looks darker. Purse the lips gently together to even out the color more.

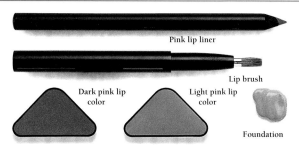

Pink lip liner

Lip brush

Dark pink lip color

Light pink lip color

Foundation

Outline just outside natural
edge of lips to emphasize
their shape

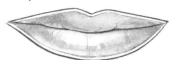

Brush on a slightly
glossy color

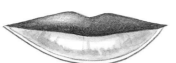

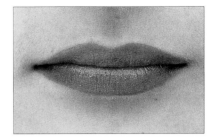

Outline along natural
edge of fuller half
of uneven lip

Outline outside
thinner half of
uneven lip

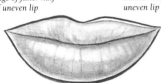

Brush on color, adding
more to thinner part of
uneven lip

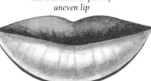

Outline lower lip

Outline top lip to
accentuate cupid's bow

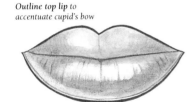

Brush on a strong,
definite color

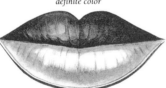

Outline outside
natural edge of lower lip

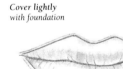

Cover lightly
with foundation

Brush on color, avoiding
pearly or glossy shades

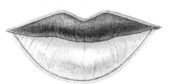

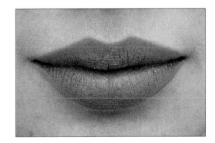

Outline inside
natural edge of lips

Cover lightly
with foundation

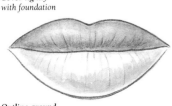

Brush a lighter color
onto darker lip

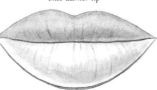

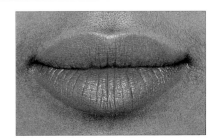

Outline around
natural edge

MANICURE

For hands to look their best, nails need to be clean and cared for. A weekly manicure will help keep them in good condition and should only take about half an hour once you have had some practice. If you do not have time to apply nail polish properly, simply buff nails with a chamois polisher to give them a natural, healthy shine. Try to use a protective, nourishing hand cream every day (see pages 110–11) and always make sure you dry your hands thoroughly each time they get wet, gently pushing back the cuticles with a towel as you do so.

── PALETTE ──

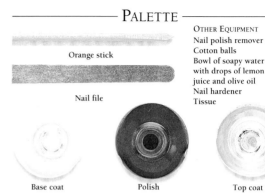

Orange stick

Nail file

OTHER EQUIPMENT
Nail polish remover
Cotton balls
Bowl of soapy water
with drops of lemon
juice and olive oil
Nail hardener
Tissue

Base coat   Polish   Top coat

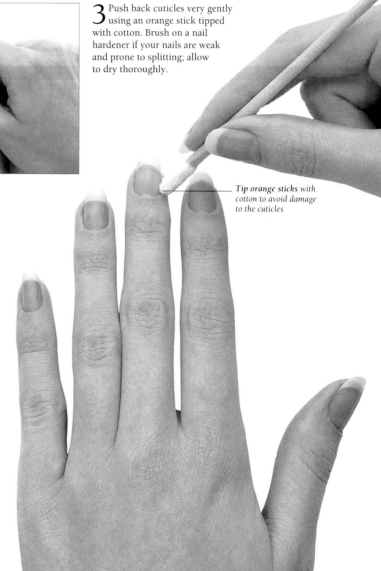

3 Push back cuticles very gently using an orange stick tipped with cotton. Brush on a nail hardener if your nails are weak and prone to splitting; allow to dry thoroughly.

Tip orange sticks with cotton to avoid damage to the cuticles

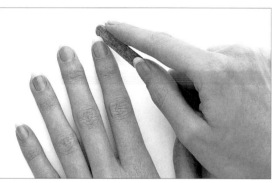

1 File nails into shape. Always file from one edge of the nail to the center, and then from the other edge back to the center. Use long, smooth strokes and never saw at the nail. File the top of the nail slightly flat if it becomes too pointed. Remove all traces of old polish using an acetone-free remover and cotton balls.

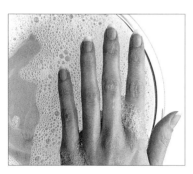

2 Soak hands for a few minutes in a bowl of soapy water to which a few drops of lemon juice and olive oil have been added; this helps to clean and soften hands at the same time. Dry thoroughly and clean away any dirt underneath the nails with an orange stick.

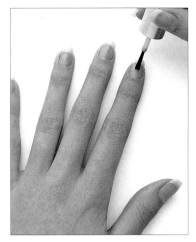

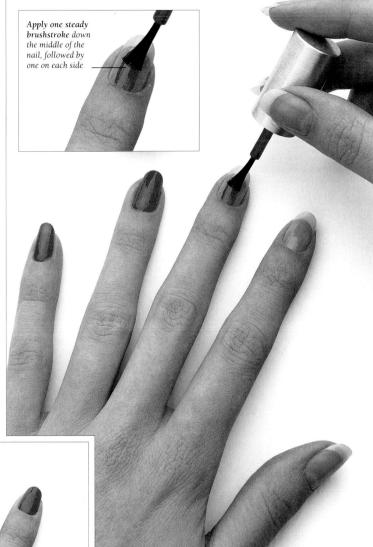

Apply one steady brushstroke down the middle of the nail, followed by one on each side

4 Lay your hand on a flat surface and brush on a base coat to prevent the nails from staining. This also strengthens nails and allows polish to be applied more smoothly. Allow to dry for a few minutes.

5 ▷Apply polish, starting with one brushstroke in the middle of the nail and then one on each side. When dry, apply a second coat of color in the same way. Carefully clear away any blobs that might have formed at the side of the nail with an orange stick tipped with cotton soaked in remover, or a small piece of tissue with remover on it. When dry, repeat with a clear top coat.

THE FINISHED EFFECT: Nails shine with beauty and health once they have been cleaned, shaped, and colored

TIPS

◆ *Calcium is said to keep nails strong and healthy; dairy products, legumes, leafy green vegetables, and dried fruit are all rich sources. However, it takes about six months for a nail to be renewed, so do not expect to see changes overnight.*

◆ *When removing polish, soak cotton balls with acetone-free remover and stroke down the nail, working from the cuticle to the tip. Do not rub or you will cause the color to streak onto the skin.*

EFFECTS FOR NAILS

DAYTIME LOOK Daytime colors should be easy to wear, such as soft reds and pinks, gentle beiges and dusky blues. First, file nails into a short, square style to create a practical, sporty effect. Apply a base coat, let dry and then give nails two coats of colored polish. Finish off with a top coat.

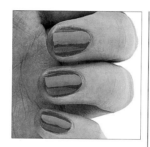

PARTY TIME This is your chance to try out those shades that you might feel afraid of wearing during the day. First, apply a base coat, then two coats of a vibrant fluorescent polish, such as this green. Add extra shine by using a sparkling silver polish on top of the main color when it is dry. Finish off with a top coat.

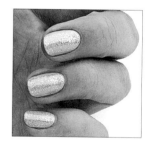

PALETTE

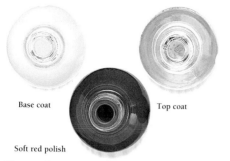

Base coat

Top coat

Soft red polish

PALETTE

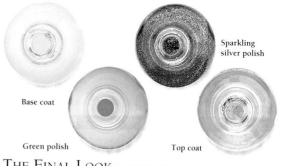

Sparkling silver polish

Base coat

Green polish

Top coat

THE FINAL LOOK

A practical, natural style based on short, square nails and a soft, easy-to-wear polish

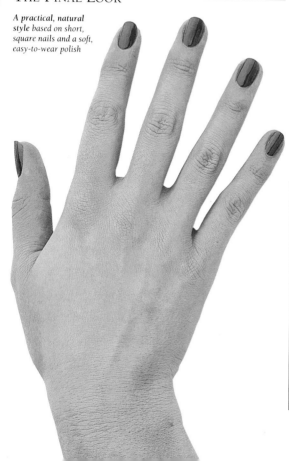

THE FINAL LOOK

Fluorescent colors are great for parties as they look so vibrant; a coat of sparkling silver polish adds the finishing touch

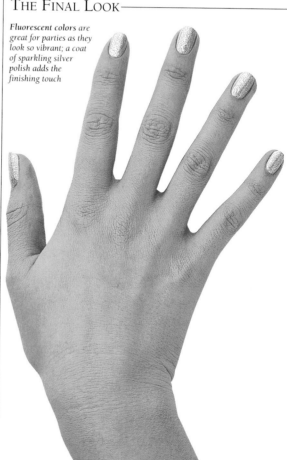

GLOSSY GLAMOUR For a grown-up, glamorous effect, choose deep, dark colors that strike a dramatic note, such as this vampish purple. First, file nails into a long, oval shape and apply a base coat. Give nails at least two coats of main polish, allowing them to dry thoroughly in between. Finish with a top coat.

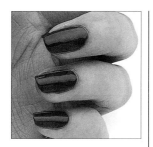

FRENCH MANICURE This is the best choice for special occasions when you want nails to look perfectly cared for, but not too loud. Apply a base coat and, when dry, cover the tips of the nails with white polish. Let dry and apply a very pale pink or peach polish over the whole nail. When dry, apply a top coat.

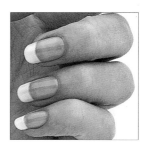

PALETTE

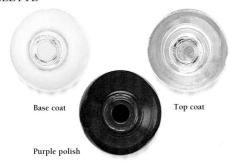

Base coat

Top coat

Purple polish

PALETTE

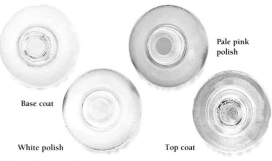

Pale pink polish

Base coat

White polish

Top coat

THE FINAL LOOK

A dark, dramatic polish gives long nails a touch of glamorous sophistication

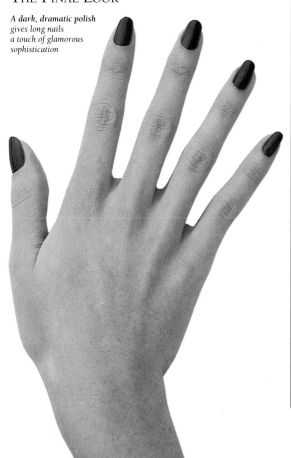

THE FINAL LOOK

A clean, fresh effect that enhances the natural shine and color of the nails

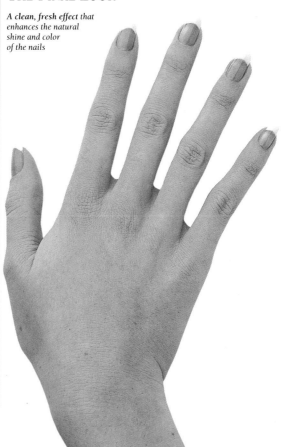

EFFECTS USING COLOR

IDEAS FOR LIGHT HAIR

Fresh and natural or sleek and sophisticated, a change of color can create very different looks.

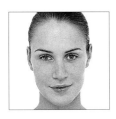

GREENS After applying foundation, brush on a light golden blusher. Cover the eye area with a pearly green shadow and use bright green on the lid. Apply bright green along the lower lash line and highlight the brow with a yellow shadow. Outline the lips with a terra-cotta lip liner and brush on a pale terra-cotta lip color.

PINKS After applying foundation, brush on a strong pink blusher, blending well. Use a pale pink pearly shadow all over the eye area and a dark rose pink shadow on the lid only. Outline the lips with a bright pink lip liner and brush on at least two coats of a strong pink lip color.

GREEN PALETTE

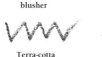
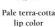
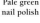

Light golden blusher

Pearly green eyeshadow

Bright green eyeshadow

Yellow eyeshadow

Pale green nail polish

Terra-cotta lip liner

Pale terra-cotta lip color

PINK PALETTE

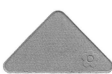
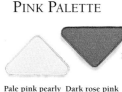

Strong pink blusher

Pale pink pearly eyeshadow

Dark rose pink eyeshadow

Base nail polish: Pink

Bright pink lip liner

Strong pink lip color

Top polish: Glittery pink

IDEAS FOR DARK HAIR

From vibrant oranges to moody blues, color can dramatically alter your appearance.

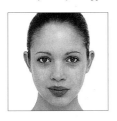

ORANGES After applying foundation, brush on a brown blusher. Cover the eye area with a pearly gold shadow and blend an orange shadow onto the lid. Use a deep orange on the socket line and a burgundy shadow along both lash lines. Outline the lips with an orange lip liner and brush on an orangey bronze lip color.

BLUES After applying foundation, brush on a light pink blusher. Cover the eye area with a pearly blue shadow and use bright blue on the lid. Continue bright blue along the lower lash line and into the inner corner. Outline the lips with a soft brown lip liner; brush on a pale terra-cotta lip color, then a touch of brown.

ORANGE PALETTE

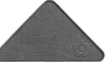

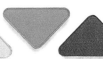

Brown blusher

Pearly gold eyeshadow

Orange eyeshadow

Deep orange eyeshadow

Burgundy eyeshadow

Burgundy nail polish

Orange lip liner

Orangey bronze lip color

BLUE PALETTE

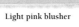
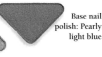
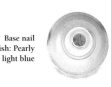

Light pink blusher

Pearly blue eyeshadow

Bright blue eyeshadow

Base nail polish: Pearly light blue

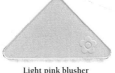

Soft brown lip liner

Pale terra-cotta lip color

Brown lip color

Top nail polish: Strong aqua

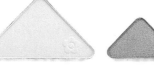

THE FINAL LOOKS

NATURAL GREENS

A blend of green and yellow eyeshadows creates a refreshing, natural look that suits a light tan

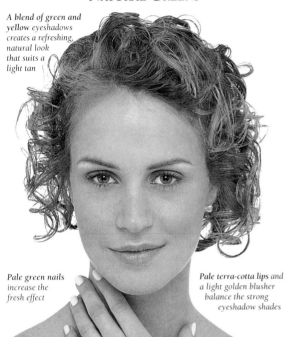

Pale green nails increase the fresh effect

Pale terra-cotta lips and a light golden blusher balance the strong eyeshadow shades

STYLISH PINKS

Based on a sleek and stylish color scheme, this smart, grown-up effect focuses on the lips

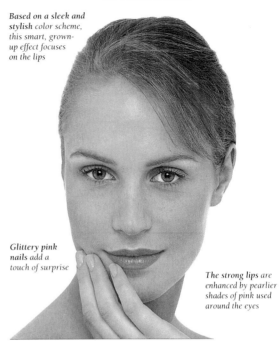

Glittery pink nails add a touch of surprise

The strong lips are enhanced by pearlier shades of pink used around the eyes

ORANGE SIZZLERS

A blend of orange eyeshadows creates a fresh, fun, and upbeat style

Bright eyeshadows are complemented by a softer orange on the lips

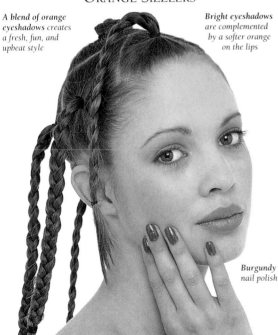

Burgundy nail polish

BOLD BLUES

A cool, moody, yet sophisticated color scheme based on a combination of soft and bright blues

Cool-toned pinky brown lips add to the dramatic, mysterious effect

Strong aqua nail polish

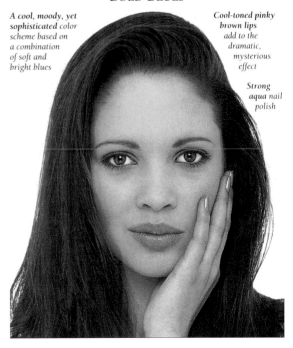

105

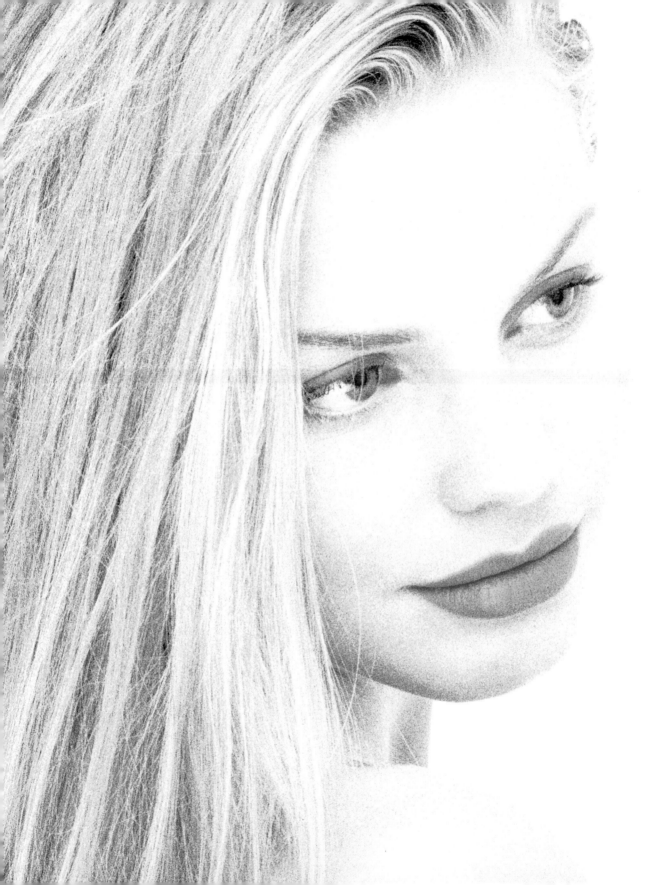

BODY-CARE PROGRAMS

Your body deserves just as much attention as your face

and should regularly be given a full range of pampering

treatments. From a deep-cleansing bathing treatment to an

all-over self-massage, the following programs

will help you tone and revitalize your body in the comfort of

your own bathroom and so shake off the stresses of everyday

life. There are also hints and tips on diet, exercise, and

relaxation, because the more you know about

how your body works, the better you can take care of it.

YOUR BODY

The more you learn about your body and how it works, the better you can take care of it and keep it looking its best. Try not to be self-conscious about your individual shape; instead, concentrate on being more body conscious, learning how to revitalize and recharge yourself through a combination of exercise, diet, and relaxation. You may also like to expand your beauty routine so that you have time to beautify your whole body with a range of pampering home treatments.

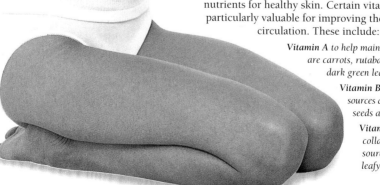

EXERCISE

EXERCISE NOT ONLY KEEPS YOU IN SHAPE, it makes you feel more relaxed and helps you sleep well and enables you to handle stress better – all of which will benefit the appearance of your skin and body. Exercise also reduces the body's fat reserves by converting them into energy and so helps improve body shape. Building an exercise program into your routine is probably one of the most positive steps you can take to enhance your body. Start with gentle activities such as walking, stretching, or swimming, and work up to five 30-minute sessions a week.

RELAXATION TECHNIQUES

ONCE A DAY, take time to relax your body and mind, and free yourself from tension. Relaxing is a skill that needs to be learned and developed; start by practicing these simple but effective techniques.

1 ◁ Abdominal breathing helps induce calmness. Place one hand on your chest and the other on your abdomen. Breathe in slowly and deeply through your nose, allowing your stomach to expand but keeping your chest still. Breathe out slowly through your nose and repeat for five to ten minutes.

2 Close your eyes and count backward from 20, saying each number silently as you breathe out. Repeat several times.

3 Shut your eyes and imagine a tranquil scene. Hold the picture in your mind for five minutes without allowing other thoughts to intrude.

DIET

EVEN THE MOST SOPHISTICATED skin-care and body treatments will not be effective if you do not feed your skin from within. Drink plenty of water (four glasses a day or more) and herbal teas to flush out toxins and prevent dehydration. Ensure that your diet contains the essential nutrients for healthy skin. Certain vitamins are thought to be particularly valuable for improving the complexion and boosting the circulation. These include:

Vitamin A to help maintain the skin's elasticity. Good sources are carrots, rutabagas, yellow or orange vegetables, and dark green leafy vegetables.

Vitamin B3 to promote healthy circulation. Good sources are grains, beans, green leafy vegetables, seeds and nuts, and fish and seafood.

Vitamin C to assist in the formation of collagen (the skin's support fibers). Good sources are citrus fruit, broccoli, green leafy vegetables, cherries, and apricots.

THE OZONE LAYER ABOVE THE EARTH no longer provides a sufficient filter to protect skin against the sun's harmful UV rays, which cause, at the very least, premature wrinkles and, at worst, an increased risk of skin cancer. Although a tan used to be associated with glowing good health, it is in fact the body's way of trying to protect against skin damage. Cells in the outer skin layer respond to sunlight by producing more of the protective pigment melanin. Dark-skinned people have more melanin; those with a fair complexion or a tendency to freckle have less and so burn more easily.

UNDERSTANDING SUN PROTECTION FACTORS

Skin that has been repeatedly damaged by sunburn is at the greatest risk of damage and also provides a poor base for makeup. Suncare and cosmetic products with a sunscreen will help protect and care for your skin, particularly if you spend a lot of time outside. The higher the SPF (sun protection factor), the longer the product will protect against sunburn. For example, as a guideline, an SPF 15 sunscreen will allow you to stay in the sun 15 times longer than you could with no protection (see the chart below), while an SPF 20 will allow you to stay 20 times longer.

SUNBLOCKS

If you want to make sure your skin hardly changes color in the sun or give exposed areas extra protection, you need to wear a sunblock. Sunblocks screen out damaging UV rays, but should also moisturize the skin. Always use a sunblock made especially for the face and a separate one for the body. A sunblock for the face will prevent tanning and freckles, but should also provide a smooth base for makeup if you intend to wear it on top. For this reason, choose a natural-colored sunblock that will not affect the color of your foundation. For best results, apply in the morning, about ten minutes after moisturizing.

SAFER TANNING

If you do want to get a tan, gradually build up the time you spend in the sun. Start off with ten minutes and add a few minutes each day. Do not sunbathe when the sun is at its strongest – usually between 11:00 a.m. and 4:00 p.m – and always wear a pair of good-quality sunglasses.

APPLYING SUNSCREEN

1 Gently rub a sunscreen with an SPF that provides the right amount of protection for your skin coloring all over your body. Reapply when necessary and always after swimming or exercise if the sunscreen is not water resistant.

2 ▷ Sensitive parts of the body, such as the shoulders, are particularly vulnerable to sunburn and may need extra protection with a sunblock, so rub onto these areas evenly.

3 After sunbathing, moisturize skin well with after-sun products to prevent it from becoming dry and peeling.

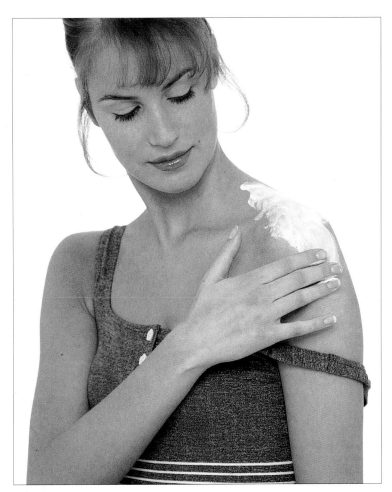

BURNING TIMES

Skin coloring		
Fair	Normal	Dark
Amount of time before burning with no protection		
10 minutes	20 minutes	30 minutes

HAND & FOOT CARE

No matter how well cared for the rest of you looks, a pair of rough, wrinkled hands will quickly ruin the effect. The skin on your hands can easily become dehydrated and damaged because it is frequently exposed to the drying effects of wind, sunshine, and water. This means that your hands can show signs of aging before other parts of your body, even your face. Their condition depends on how well you take care of them. Feet, too, tend to be forgotten, yet when your feet are feeling comfortable and relaxed, it shows immediately in how you walk and carry your body. Like hands, feet deserve special attention in order to relieve tiredness and prevent a buildup of rough skin.

MOISTURIZING YOUR HANDS

A DAILY TREATMENT with a moisturizing hand cream or lotion will help keep the skin soft and supple. It also forms a barrier against the elements and harsh cleansing agents. The best time to moisturize your hands is after an evening bath, when the skin will be most receptive. For extra protection, use a hand cream with an added SPF (see page 109).

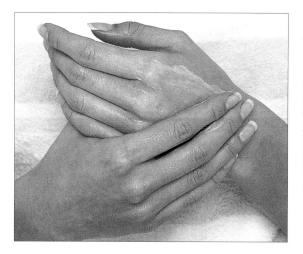

1 Wash and dry hands (for a complete cleansing treatment, see page 100).

2 ◁ Massage hand cream thoroughly into both hands, gently pushing back the nail cuticles with a towel as you do so; do not push with the tip of the nail as this can cause the other nail to become ridged. Massaging helps stimulate circulation and can also alleviate tension and stiffness.

PAMPERING YOUR FEET

FEET ARE THE HARDEST-WORKING parts of the body, but we rarely make time to give them the attention they need. A weekly pampering pedicure and massage is the answer and will leave feet feeling refreshed and ready for action.

1 Soak feet in a bowl of hot water for about ten minutes. Add two to three drops of essential oil of lavender for an even more relaxing effect.

2 Dry the feet. Clip the toenails across and file smooth.

3 Rub feet with an exfoliating body scrub, paying particular attention to any rough skin that may have formed on the heels and the balls of the feet. Wash off all traces of exfoliator and dry the feet thoroughly.

4 ▷ Support the foot with one hand by placing your thumb on the sole and your fingers on the top. Use the other hand to massage a cooling foot lotion or an overall body moisturizer into the foot. Start at the base of each toe and work down the foot, making small circular movements with your thumb and forefinger.

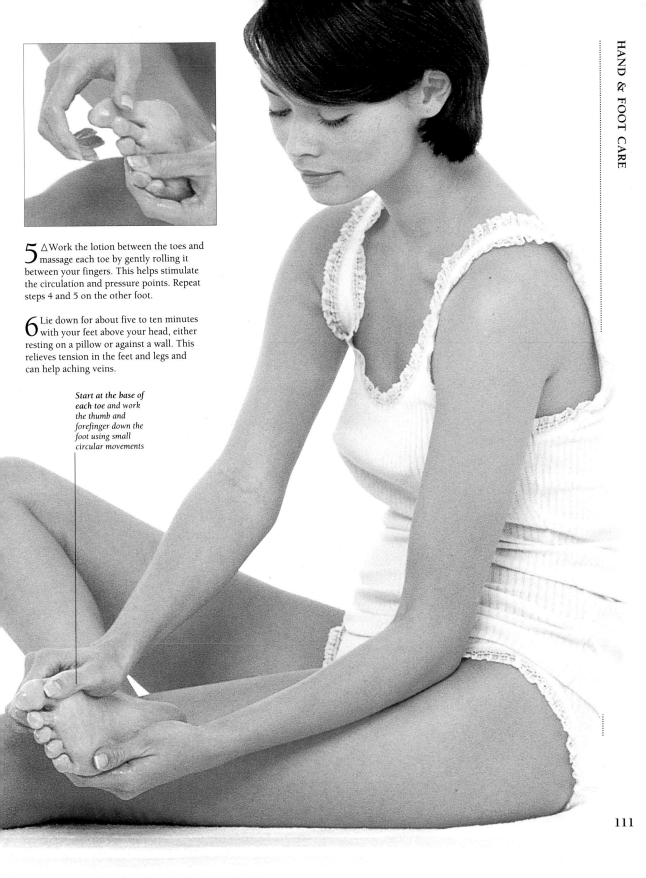

5 △Work the lotion between the toes and massage each toe by gently rolling it between your fingers. This helps stimulate the circulation and pressure points. Repeat steps 4 and 5 on the other foot.

6 Lie down for about five to ten minutes with your feet above your head, either resting on a pillow or against a wall. This relieves tension in the feet and legs and can help aching veins.

Start at the base of each toe and work the thumb and forefinger down the foot using small circular movements

BATH TREATMENT

Think of your bathroom as a private room where you can escape from the pressures of modern life, and as a therapy center where you can completely relax and indulge yourself at the end of the day. A long soak in a warm bath in the evening not only relieves tension, stimulates the circulation, and softens the skin, it will soothe tired, aching joints and open the pores ready for moisturizing. If it helps you relax, read or cover your eyes with a pair of eyepads and listen to some calming music while you are soaking in the bath. Always make sure that you have a warm towel and bathrobe ready to wrap yourself in when you have finished your bath treatment.

CLEANSING THE BODY

1 Fill the bath with warm water, but do not make it too hot as this could raise your heartbeat and make it difficult for you to sleep later. Add some scented bath crystals or bath oil to the water; choosing a product that contains sea minerals or salts will add to the feeling of creating a spa in your own bathroom. Test that the temperature of the water is comfortable before stepping into the bath.

2 Lie back in the warm water, immersing as much of your body as possible. Close your eyes – or put on eyepads – and relax for at least ten minutes. If you find it hard to switch off, try practicing the relaxation techniques on page 108.

3 ◁ Using a pair of bath mitts, concentrate on washing your body from top to toe, working from the feet upward. Pour a little body shampoo onto the mitten for a deep-cleansing treatment. Use gentle circular movements and take time to focus on pampering yourself in your own private sanctuary.

4 Soak for another ten minutes, adding more warm water if necessary, and meanwhile work on the acupressure points on the soles of the feet and on the lower legs as shown opposite.

5 Rinse off excessive lather and dry yourself thoroughly with a warm towel. Massage a non-oily body lotion all over the body (see pages 114–15).

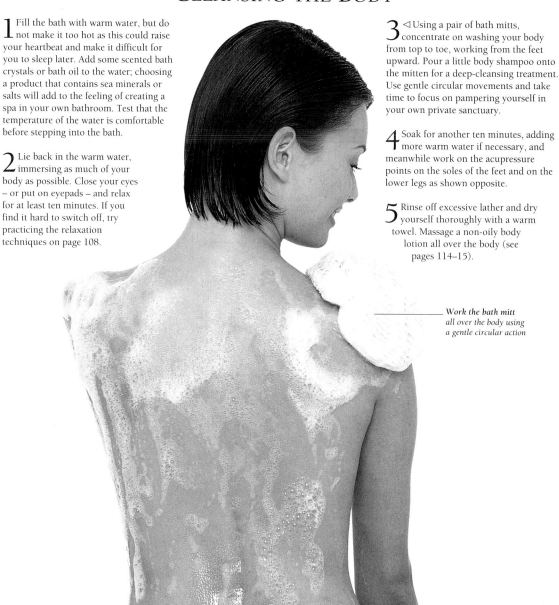

Work the bath mitt all over the body using a gentle circular action

ACUPRESSURE POINTS

ACUPRESSURE COULD BE THOUGHT OF as acupuncture without the needles. It is basically a self-help technique in which the fingers are used to apply pressure to particular points, which are thought to relieve pain or promote positive health benefits by stimulating the flow of energy through the body. In Japan, it is known as shiatsu, or finger massage. There are about 600 different acupressure points found all over the body; they can often feel a little more sensitive than the surrounding area and can be located by their slight indentation. Pressure is applied with the fingers for a few seconds at a time; the process can be repeated three or four times at each spot.

1 Press the acupressure point on the sole of the foot, marked point A right. Release after a few seconds and repeat three or four times. This is sometimes known as the "gushing spring" point and helps any kidney-related problems as well as stimulating a flow of energy throughout the body.

2 Press the acupressure point on the back of your ankle, marked point B right. Release after a few seconds and repeat three or four times. This helps improve digestion and can help relieve backache.

3 Apply pressure to the acupressure points on the front of the lower leg, working upward from the lowest point. Release after a few seconds and repeat three or four times. This improves blood circulation and relieves tiredness in the legs.

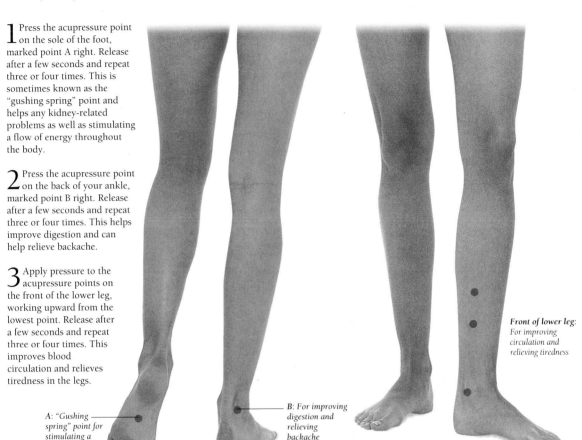

Front of lower leg: *For improving circulation and relieving tiredness*

A: "Gushing spring" point for stimulating a flow of energy

B: For improving digestion and relieving backache

BODY BRUSHING

FOR EXTRA-CLEAN SKIN, brush your body every day before you get into the bath or shower. This will help slough off dead skin cells and other forms of surface dirt. Dry skin brushing is also thought to be effective in the battle against cellulite (see page 117) as it boosts the lymphatic drainage system into action, breaking down toxins that have become trapped in the fat cells. It should take about five minutes to brush your whole body, and afterward your skin will feel smooth but invigorated; if your skin begins to feel sore and rough, you are probably brushing too hard.

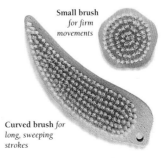

Small brush *for firm movements*

Curved brush *for long, sweeping strokes*

Use a natural-bristled brush and make long sweeping movements in the direction of the heart. Sweep the soles of the feet first, then work toward the knees. Use firmer, circular movements on the thighs, hips and buttocks, but be more gentle over the stomach and breasts. Use a long-handled brush to reach down the back.

113

DAILY FIRMING MASSAGE

Massage has long been known to relax muscles and reduce stress. It is also thought to improve circulation and cleanse the body of toxins. But, best of all, it makes you feel good. Always wait about ten minutes after finishing a bath treatment before starting a massage to allow your energy levels to return to normal. Work smoothly and rhythmically to leave yourself feeling as relaxed as possible, and use a massage oil or your normal body moisturizer.

1 Sit in a comfortable position. Apply some oil or moisturizer to your hands, wrap them around one calf to spread the oil, and massage upward using a circular motion. Repeat the movement five times and then work on the other leg.

2 Place eight fingers on the middle of the calf and pull upward. This stimulates the lymphatic system. Repeat the process on the other leg.

3 Grab the fat on one thigh with one hand, gently pull upward, and twist the flesh, applying pressure with your thumb. Repeat with the other hand, alternating the action for about five minutes. Repeat on the other thigh.

4 Massage the arms to release tension in the shoulders. Using one hand, stroke firmly up the other arm, from the wrist to the shoulder. Repeat on the other arm.

5 ◁ Use a kneading movement all the way up the arm, concentrating on any fleshy points. Repeat on the other arm.

6 Lie on your back and knead all over the abdomen using your fingers and thumbs. Roll onto one side to repeat the strokes on your hips and buttocks. Repeat on the other side.

7 Stand up, loosely clench your fists, and pummel your buttocks and hips as fast as possible. (As this is a vigorous action, you might want to omit it if you are doing the massage just before going to bed.)

Knead up and down the arm, concentrating on any fleshy points

Sit as comfortably as possible

SPECIAL TONING MASSAGE

ONCE A WEEK, or when you have more time to spare, extend your daily massage to work further on key areas such as the waist, arms, and legs. These are points where fat can easily build up and muscles lose their tone. Start by pinching the fat as if you were kneading, concentrating on the points shown below, then massage firmly around the point for about five minutes. This helps boost blood circulation to these key areas, as well as stimulating the lymphatic drainage system. As with the daily massage, either use your body moisturizer or a special massage oil.

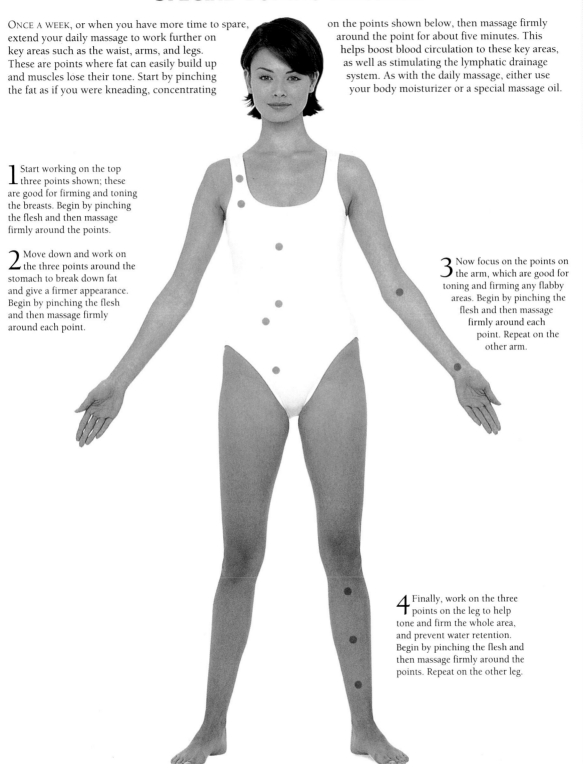

1 Start working on the top three points shown; these are good for firming and toning the breasts. Begin by pinching the flesh and then massage firmly around the points.

2 Move down and work on the three points around the stomach to break down fat and give a firmer appearance. Begin by pinching the flesh and then massage firmly around each point.

3 Now focus on the points on the arm, which are good for toning and firming any flabby areas. Begin by pinching the flesh and then massage firmly around each point. Repeat on the other arm.

4 Finally, work on the three points on the leg to help tone and firm the whole area, and prevent water retention. Begin by pinching the flesh and then massage firmly around the points. Repeat on the other leg.

BODY SCRUB

Two or three times a week, give yourself a special treat and use a gentle exfoliating scrub or cream all over the body. This will slough off dull surface cells to give the skin a finer texture and better color, as well as boosting sluggish circulation. Exfoliation also softens those areas prone to hard skin, such as the heels, knees, and elbows. And sloughing off dead skin makes it easier for moisturizers to be absorbed. Body scrubs should be slightly rougher than facial scrubs, but do not use on vulnerable areas, such as the neck, the underarms, and the backs of the knees.

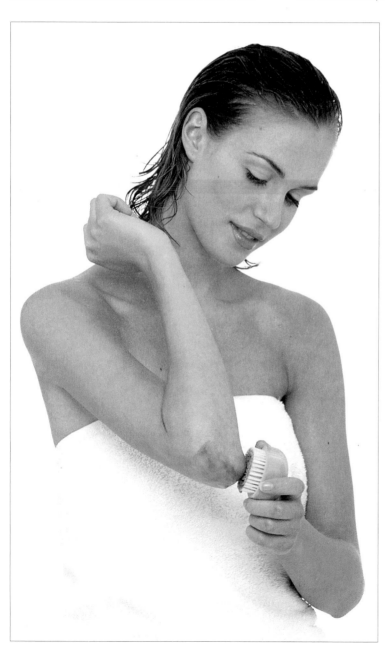

1 When your skin is still moist after showering, gently massage a little scrub into the areas that are prone to cellulite: the hips, buttocks, and thighs. Work on each area for about two minutes but do not rub too hard, as this will cause skin to become red and dry.

2 ◁ Now concentrate on the parts of the body where hard skin is most likely to develop, such as the elbows, the front of the knees, and the heels, rubbing the scrub in with a small body brush.

3 Shower off all traces of the scrub, using the water to massage in circular movements over the thighs, hips, buttocks, and breasts. If you are feeling brave, finish by showering with cold water.

4 Gently rub dry with a firm towel and then massage a moisturizing body lotion over your whole body (see page 114).

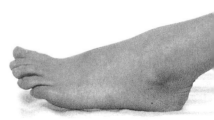

CELLULITE TREATMENT

Cellulite is that unattractive "orange-peel" effect caused by the dimpled skin that often develops on the thighs, buttocks, and hips. More than just a sign of being overweight, it is a signal that waste, toxins, and fat deposits are building up in these areas. Anyone can develop cellulite, even thin people. Localized massage is one of the best ways to treat cellulite as it helps to drain away waste, as well as making the skin look smoother and tighter. However, any exercise that works the upper legs, such as cycling and jogging, will also help.

TONING PROBLEM AREAS

1 Using a special anti-cellulite oil, massage oil, or body lotion, knead the hips and buttocks by squeezing and lifting the flesh with one hand and then the other. Work all over these areas wherever you can pick up enough flesh.

2 Apply more oil if necessary and stroke smoothly from above the knee to the top of the thigh and from the back of the knee to the buttocks. Repeat on the other leg.

3 ▷ Knead the thigh from the knee to the top of the leg, front and back, using deep movements to squeeze and lift the flesh. This stimulates blood circulation and lymphatic drainage. Repeat on the other leg.

4 Wrap both hands around the leg just above the knee and pull the flesh up toward the top of the thigh. Repeat on the other leg.

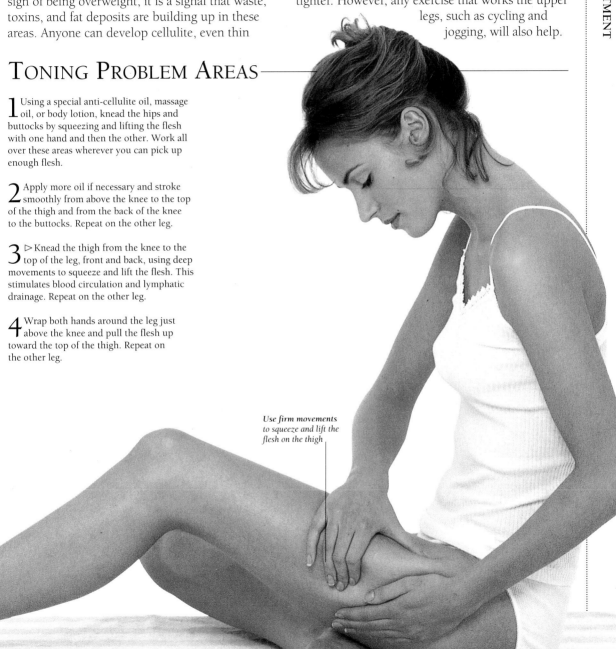

Use firm movements to squeeze and lift the flesh on the thigh

117

INDEX

ACKNOWLEDGMENTS

AUTHOR'S ACKNOWLEDGMENTS

I must thank Dorling Kindersley for the marvelously talented and professional team they produced to work with me on this bumper book, including Louise Elliott for her amazing ability to rationalize magic; Michele Walker for her infallible eye; Helen Diplock for her sure-fire design anticipation of the whole book; Carole Ash for pure, clear art direction; Susannah Marriott for ensuring beautiful, simple editing throughout; and everyone else who was involved in the production of the book. So incredibly in unison were we that I started to feel deprived of a good fight and to look for trouble myself. But no – the whole book floated through on a tide of good fortune, sound sense, and fun, helped along by Maureen Barrymore's delicious photographic lunches.

I would also like to thank Maureen Barrymore for her wonderful photographs that so clearly love the stylish dash of makeup as much as naked beauty; Dave King for the clarity and punch of his step-by-step photographs; Cathy Lomax for her charmingly funky good taste that so appeals to me; Vidal Sassoon for letting us have Billi Currie, Peter Gray, and Ben Skervin to work their spells on the hair styles; all the models for being so generous with their beauty; and manager Angela Watson and consultant Sarah Stent at the Mary Quant Colour Shop for casting their professional eye over the book and for offering the most satisfying tips, on everything from skin-care to applying makeup.

PUBLISHER'S ACKNOWLEDGMENTS

Dorling Kindersley would like to thank the following: Clare Maxwell-Hudson for checking massage sequences on pages 68–71 and 108–117; Angela and Sarah at the Mary Quant shop for their boundless patience and enthusiasm throughout the whole project; Sara Mulholland-Wright at Profile for all her help and advice in casting and booking the right models; Nasim Mawji for research and product testing.

Photographers: Maureen Barrymore pages 6–15, 18–27, 32 bottom left and top right, 34, 35 top, 36, 37 top, 56–57, 72–73, 98 bottom, 104–117. Dave King pages 28–31, 32 bottom right, 33, 37 bottom, 58–71, 74–93, 96–103. Martyn Thompson pages 16–17, 32 top left, 35 bottom, 94–95.

DK Photographic Studio: Steve Gorton pages 10–25 palettes, 38–55 beauty-care products, 80–83 palettes, 86–101 palettes. Sarah Ashun pages 34–37 palettes, 74–79 palettes, 84–85 palettes, 102–5 palettes; as well as assisting Steve.

Models: Audrey Drake, Caroline Iuel Brockdorff, Francesca Howie, Gitte Rosengaard, Katie Tomlinson, Mary Grimes, Rachel Clarke, Stephanie Green, Susan Lelis, and Vanessa Franco at Profile. Gillian McConnachie, Karen Elson, Mayumi Cabrera, Terri Seymour and Wendy New at Models 1. Jo Branfoot, Michelle Mason, Oxana Popkova, and Sonia Gardner at Select. Donna Astbury, Holly Venn, Julia May and Natasha Brice at Storm. Wendi Anthony at IMG Models. Kanako Morishit at Oriental Casting Agency. Charlotte Saunders and Kara O'Neill at 2 Management. Sara Francis at Freddie's. Shoko Kai. Joanna Aitkens.

Makeup: Cathy Lomax at Debbie Walters except: Jane Bradley at The Worx pages 58–62, 98 center, 108–117. Fay Leith pages 63, 64–71, 78–79, 82–83, as well as assisting Cathy. Special thanks to Cathy for consultancy work and editorial input on pages 10–25 and 74–105.

Hair: Billi Currie, Peter Gray, and Ben Skervin, at Vidal Sassoon; Alison Johnson for booking arrangements.

Clothes and makeup: from the Mary Quant Colour Shop, 3 Ives Street, London SW3 2NE. Jewelry on pages 20–21 from Butler & Wilson.

Photographic retouching: Ken McMahon at Pelican Graphics.

Product retouching: Tim Weare & Partners.

Artwork: Karen Cochrane for arrow artworks throughout the book, as well as face-shape artworks on pages 84–85.

Illustrations: Julie Carpenter for pages 29, 30–31, 94–95 and 98–99.

Index: Kate Chapman